RIGHTS AND RESPONSIBILITIES IN MODERN MEDICINE

The Second Volume in a Series on Ethics, Humanism, and Medicine

RIGHTS AND RESPONSIBILITIES IN MODERN MEDICINE

The Second Volume in a Series on Ethics, Humanism, and Medicine

Proceedings of the 1979—1980 Conferences on
Ethics, Humanism, and Medicine at the
University of Michigan, Ann Arbor

Editor
MARC D. BASSON

ALAN R. LISS, INC., NEW YORK

Library of Congress Cataloging in Publication Data

Main entry under title:

Rights and responsibilities in modern medicine.

(Progress in clinical and biological research; 50)
Includes bibliographical references and index.
1. Medical ethics – Congresses. I. Basson, Marc D.
II. Committee on Ethics, Humanism, and Medicine.
III. Series. [DNLM: 1. Ethics, Medical – Congresses.
2. Patient advocacy – Congresses. W1 PR668e v. 50/
W 50 C7415 1979–80r]
R724.R496   174′.2   80-29391
ISBN 0-8451-0050-5

Contents

Marc D. Basson is currently a fourth year medical student at
the University of Michigan. He received his A.B. from the
University of Michigan in "Philosophy of Medicine" and
subsequently did a student internship at the Institute for
Society, Ethics and the Life Sciences. He founded and is
currently the Director of the Committee on Ethics, Humanism,
and Medicine. In addition to editing the proceedings of the
Committee's first three conferences (also published by Alan
R. Liss, Inc.), he has published in The Journal of Medicine
and Philosophy.

Tom Beauchamp is a professor of philosophy at Georgetown
University and Senior Research Scholar at the Kennedy
Institute for Bioethics. In addition to a number of an-
thologies on bioethical issues, he has himself published a
wide variety of materials on matters philosophical and
bioethical. These include *Principles of Biomedical Ethics*
(with James Childress) and the article on "Paternalism" in
the *Encyclopedia of Bioethics*. He is a staff philospher for
the National Institutes of Health.

Eric Cassell is a professor of public health and a practicing
internist affiliated with Cornell University. He is a
Fellow of the Institute for Society, Ethics and the Life
Sciences. The list of his organizational affiliations is
long, and his writings on bioethics are equally impressive.
Most relevant to this paper is his work on problems of
doctor-patient communication, autonomy, and medical paternalism. He has also presented papers on "Errors in Medicine"
and "The Patient's Right to Refuse Treatment" as well as
"The Patient's Autonomy in Medicine."

Bennett Cohen is Director of the Unit for Laboratory Animal
Medicine at the University of Michigan Medical School and
holds both a D.V.M. and a Ph.D. in Physiology. He pioneer-
ed the development of the notion that laboratory animal care
needs to be carefully supervised by a specialist in this
field as well as by experimenters. He serves as a frequent
site visitor and consultant to the NIH on grant proposals
and has assisted in the development of numerous proposals
and codes for care of laboratory animals both here and
abroad. He serves on the Program Committee of the Inter-

national Committee on Laboratory Animals General Assembly in
the Netherlands.

Norman Daniels is a professor of philosophy at Tufts University
and a co-director of the study group on Justice and Resource
Allocation of the Institute for Society, Ethics and the Life
Sciences. He has published extensively on theories of
justice and in the field of medical ethics. Among his
recent publications are *Reading Rawls*, an anthology on the
nature of justice, and *Justice and Health Care Delivery*.

A. Edward Doudera received his J.D. from Suffolk University
School of Law in 1978. He is presently Executive Director
of the American Society of Law & Medicine, which is head-
quartered in Boston. Mr. Doudera also serves as Managing
Editor of the Medicolegal News and as Executive Editor of
the American Journal of Law & Medicine. Before joining the
society, Mr. Doudera was Associate Administrator for Research at Tufts-New England Medical Center.

Meredith Eiker is a graduate of the University of Michigan
and received a Master's degree in Public Health from Yale.
She has had extensive experience in hospital administration
and medical education and previously served on the Wayne
State University medical faculty. She has worked with the
Committee on Ethics, Humanism, and Medicine on several
projects. Ms. Eiker is presently Staff Assistant to the
Director at the Ann Arbor Veteran's Administration Medical
Center.

Faith Fitzgerald is assistant professor of medicine and
Director of Medical Student Teaching Programs at the University of Michigan Medical School. A practicing clinician
as well as an educator, she has long been concerned with
problems of medical ethics.

Norman Fost received his M.D. from Yale and his M.P.H. from
Harvard. He completed his internship and residency at Johns
Hopkins and then did a fellowship at Harvard in the Kennedy
Program for Law, Medicine, and Ethics. He is currently
Director of the Program in Medical Ethics, Chairman of the
Committee for the Protection of Human Subjects, and Assoc-
iate Professor of Pediatrics at the University of Wisconsin
School of Medicine.

Doreen Ganos has completed her undergraduate training at the
University of Michigan, and is currently a medical student
there. She has been a member of the Committee on Ethics,
Humanism, and Medicine for two years, and serves as Director
for Publicity and Registration for the Committee.

Ann Dudley Goldblatt graduated from Harvard Law School in
1961 and holds an advanced law degree from the University of
Chicago. She has taught medical ethics and medical law in
the Philosophy Department of DePaul University and at the
University of Chicago. Her teaching at Chicago has been at
both the undergraduate level and the Pritzker School of
Medicine. She previously worked in the field of public
policy litigation and has done extensive volunteer work at
Children's Memorial Hospital in Chicago.

Stanley Hauerwas is a professor of theology at the University
of Notre Dame who has been primarily concerned with basic
methodological issues in theological ethics. He has, however,
published a number of essays in the field of bioethics.
With degrees in theology and philosophy from Yale, and his
background in bioethical issues, he is uniquely qualified to
look at the issue of rational suicide from a very special
point of view.

Rachel Lipson is a student at the University of Michigan
Medical School. She has been working on the Committee for
Ethics, Humanism, and Medicine since its inception in 1978,
and is currently the Committee's Program Director.

Jerome Motto is a professor of psychiatry at the University
of California School of Medicine at San Francisco and
Associate Director of the Psychiatric Consultation Service
at the UCSF Medical Center. He has had an active interest
in the clinical aspects of depressive and suicidal states
for the past 24 years and has an impressive list of publications and activities to testify to his expertise. Among his
distinguished service to scholarly societies has been tenure
as President and Chairman of the Ethics Committee of the
American Association of Suicidology.

Carl Pursell has been involved in politics and government
first on the local and then state levels and now as a United
States Congressman. He has won a great deal of recognition
and several awards for his efforts towards budget-trimming.
He has long been interested in funding for education and, at

the time this paper was written, served on the House of Representatives HEW Appropriations Committee.

Tom Regan is currently a professor of philosophy at North Carolina State University. He was among the first to seriously espouse the notion that animals might have rights and to ask what implications these rights might have for our dietary and experimental practices. He has published numerous papers on this subject and along with Peter Singer has edited an anthology entitled *Animal Rights and Human Obligations*.

John N. Sheagren received his M.D. from Columbia University and trained at the Massachusetts General Hospital. After doing research at the National Institute of Health, he served as Chief of the Howard University Medical Service and then as Acting Chairman of the George Washington University Department of Medicine before moving to the University of Michigan in 1977. He now serves as a professor of internal medicine at the University of Michigan Medical School and as Chief of the Medical Service at the Ann Arbor Veteran's Administration Medical Center.

George Sher is a professor of philosophy at the University of Vermont and has taught courses there including "Philosophical Problems in Medicine" and "Justice and Equality". He has written several papers on questions of justice and desert and is a frequent contributor to *Philosophy and Public Affairs*.

David Smith is currently Chairman of the Department of Religious Studies at Indiana University and has been affiliated with both the Kennedy Institute for Bioethics and the Hastings Institute for Society, Ethics and the Life Sciences. He has been interested in medical ethics for many years, writing and teaching on the subject for his colleagues and for health professionals. He has been particularly active in thinking through ethical issues surrounding death and dying and has written numerous papers in this field.

Stephen Stich is currently on the faculty of the University of Maryland, and was a member of the Department of Philosophy at the University of Michigan for many years. He is most well known for his work on issues relating to recombinant DNA research, but he has taught and written widely on many ethical questions. He was exposed to other countries'

health care systems in 1977 as a Fulbright Senior Research
Scholar at Bristol, England. He has also spent one month
lecturing in Israel and some additional time in West Germany.

PREFACE

Marc D. Basson

Director, CEHM
University of Michigan
Ann Arbor, Michigan

The Committee on Ethics, Humanism, and Medicine was
founded in 1978 by students in the Integrated Premedical-
Medical Program at the University of Michigan because of
concern that the discipline of medical ethics was insuf-
ficiently accessible to the students and practitioners of
medicine and allied health care fields who most needed it.
We felt that something was needed to connect the occasional
lecture or journal article on bioethics with the clinical
situations in which ethical dilemmas arise. Furthermore, we
felt that while many different sorts of people had been
reflecting on questions of medical ethics there was insufficient communication between them. Philosophers tend to
write mostly in philosophy journals, lawyers in law reviews,
and theologians in their own periodicals. The doctors who
directly experience and must resolve problems of medical
ethics every day rarely read any of these, for they are too
busy trying to keep up with the never-ending flow of new
medical knowledge. These physicians present their own
thoughts about medical ethics in journals rarely perused by
members of these other disciplines.

Thus, we designed our first conference in 1978 with
three firm beliefs which have not changed subsequently.
First, theoretical teaching in ethics must be supplemented
by practical ethical decision-making for maximal impact.
Second, doctors and other health professionals have much to
learn from the more theoretically sophisticated philosophers,
lawyers, and theologians. Third, these same health professionals have much to offer in return from the richness of
their clinical experience.

These three principles determined the structure of our
conferences. Each topic is introduced by two speakers who
attempt to sketch their own general principles in dealing
with the issue in question and to suggest some of the
viewpoints that others have argued for. One of these
speakers is generally a clinician whose professional work
forces him to resolve questions like those being discussed.
The other is most typically a philosopher or lawyer who can
bring a more theoretical perspective to bear. After the
speakers' initial presentations, the conference participants
are divided into small groups of ten to twelve people each,
preselected to provide for maximal diversity. These groups
are charged with attempting to evolve a unanimous position
on the issues raised by the case presented in their programs,
to "solve" the case together. They are given approximately
ninety minutes. Rarely does a group actually emerge with a
consensus; but in attempting this, each group member must
clarify his own thinking and strive to understand that of
his fellow participants. After the small discussion groups,
participants reconvene to compare notes, ask questions of
the speakers, and continue their debates.

We have attempted to attract an audience in keeping
with our views about the importance of interdisciplinary
communication in matters of medical ethics, for the small
group discussion format makes each participant simultaneously
a resource person for the others. Physicians and members of
the other health care fields (public health, nursing, social
work, etc.) mingle with philosophers, lawyers, and theologians. Many of our participants are Univeristy of Michigan
faculty or faculty from other Midwestern universities.
Others are practicing physicians and allied health care
specialists from the Detroit metropolitan area. Finally,
about half are students at the University of Michigan or
other nearby schools, mostly medical students but with
significant representations of philosophy, public health,
nursing, social work, and law in addition to interested
undergraduates.

The proceedings of the first three conferences have
already been published by Alan R. Liss, Inc. as Volume 38 of
the "Progress in Clinical and Biological Research" series
under the title Ethics, Humanism, and Medicine. This volume
contains the proceedings of the fourth and fifth conferences.

Although the Committee has expanded in numbers and

diversified in background since 1977, it remains a student
organization. It is by no means a small task for a group of
students to run conferences such as these, and immense
credit must go to those who have helped us in this effort.
More have helped than we could possibly list here.

Funding for the Fourth and Fifth Conferences was
supplied by the Collegiate Institute for Values and Science,
Dr. Carolyne K. Davis, the Integrated Premedical-Medical
Program, the Jensen Foundation, Dr. Charles G. Overberger,
the Rackham School of Graduate Studies, the School of
Medicine, the School of Nursing and the School of Public
Health, all at the University of Michigan. The School of
Public Health also made the Thomas Francis Jr. Building
available to us for our conferences.

Among the University staff who helped us were Carl
Cohen, who was always ready with a helpful suggestion for
speaker-selection or an apt turn of phrase; and Ed Goldman,
on whom we could always count for legal background. Meredith
Eiker was a valuable resource person for public policy
material and provided information for the Right to Health
Care case in addition to speaking on Cost Effectiveness.
Holly Goldman and Peter Railton often provided helpful
suggestions as to speakers or topics and also helped us
train facilitators to move the small discussion groups
along. Dr. Terence Davies, Dr. Carolyne K. Davis, Dr. Errol
Erlandson, Dr. John Gronvall, Dr. Marcia Liepman, Mr.
Douglas Peters, Dr. Robert Reed, Dr. Richard Remington, Dr.
Dietrich Roloff, Dr. James Taren, and Dr. Myron Wegman all
provided valuable encouragement and guidance.

Special thanks are due to Marjorie Barritt, Alice
Cohen, Helen Ferran, Shirley Martin, Aurelia Navarro, and
Janice Wizorek, all of whom have been very enthusiastic
about the CEHM project and who have helped us greatly in
their various capacities. Aurelia Navarro and Janice
Wizorek in particular put in many long hours transcribing
and typing so that these proceedings could become a reality.

Researching topics and writing cases for them frequently
demand a great deal of expertise. In addition to those
cited above, special mention must be made of Dr. Bennett
Cohen, who wrote a good deal of the case for the Animal
Rights topic on which he subsequently spoke, and Dr. Faith
Fitzgerald, who drafted the case on which she spoke.

The students who worked on these conferences were many and we can only list a few. Rachel Lipson served ably as Conference Coordinator for the Fourth Conference and as Program Director for the Fifth. She also substantially contributed to the production of this volume, writing some of the ancillary material and helping to coordinate the typing effort. Doreen Ganos has been the Director for Publicity and Registration since CEHM was founded and also contributed to the notes in this volume. Nancy Gamburd was Director for Programming this year and helped draft the Government Funding for Elective Abortions case. She also worked on the reference lists. Sandeep Shekar worked on publicity and registration for the Fourth Conference and acted as Assistant Director for Publicity and Registration for the Fifth. Mary Johnson and Steve Teplinsky acted as Associate Directors for the Fourth Conference. Russ Herschelmann, Jonathan Oppenheimer, Anthony So and John Wallbillich also contributed greatly to the success of these conferences. Ann Minckler helped train the facilitators for the small groups for the Fifth Conference. Other students who have helped include Chuck Alejos, Vivek Allada, Mary Fox, Rahul Sanghvi, Deborah Weisbeski, and Laurie Winkelman.

Fourth Conference on
Ethics, Humanism, and Medicine
November 10, 1979

INTRODUCTION TO THE FOURTH CONFERENCE: ON RIGHTS

Marc D. Basson

Director, CEHM
University of Michigan
Ann Arbor, Michigan

Good morning and welcome to the conference.

Discussing today's topics with fellow committee
members several weeks ago, I noticed that virtually no
argument was presented without some kind of appeal to
rights. We talked about rights to health care, rights to
justice, animal rights, rights to life and rights to know.
I almost never heard that it was wrong to do this or
proper to do that without someone's rights being offered
as a justification.

Rights pervade contemporary moral discourse. In
addition to more "traditional" sorts of rights, recent
public policy debates have touched on rights to die (Heifetz,
1975), rights to food, nonsmoker's rights to clean air,
rights to act foolishly (In re Yetter, 1973), and even a
legally recognized right to enjoy sunshine (Editors,
1976). Perhaps the most bizarre instance I have encountered
involved miners on Fuji who claimed a right to a sex break
(Editors, 1976).

Now, I don't find it particularly strange that people
should want to have or to do any of these things, or even
that people should mount moral arguments in favor of these
things being permitted them. But it seems as if in the
past one would have said, for instance, "I want to breathe
clean air" or even "You ought not breathe smoke in my
face" without bringing up rights.

Are we suddenly recognizing rights that were intrinsic

to personhood all along? Or are we creating new rights by mutual agreement as some have suggested (Macklin, 1976)? Or are people simply misunderstanding the nature of rights, confusing "I want very badly" with "I have a right to"?

There may well be some truth to all of these possibilities, and I do not propose to tell you where rights really come from or what they really are. I don't know. Of course, I have some ideas about the matter, but my intuitions are not necessarily more or less likely to be "the truth" than yours, if indeed such a "truth" exists and any of us has reasoned to it.

One major problem, I think, is that the notion of a "right" means different things depending on who uses it and the circumstances in which it is used. Consider: "I have a right to be heard." "I have a right to a college education." "I have a right to live where I please." What I would like to do in the next few minutes is to discuss some of the things we might mean by "rights" and some of the ways philosophers distinguish among them; a differential diagnosis, as it were, of what it means to say that someone has a right.

First, rights language can be legal or moral in character, and we must distinguish between these. Legal rights language simply reports on the applicability of a given law to the case in question. Our protagonist in the Right to Health Care case is a veteran and has been granted a legal right to health care by our government. He has this legal right regardless of the circumstances of his case, just because the law says so. Now he has been given this legal right for a reason, because the government felt indebted to those who fought to preserve our society, and this debt may give us reason to say that he has a moral right as well. Or he may have a moral right because everyone has such a moral right. Or he may have a moral right to fair treatment under the law which endows him with the moral right to health care after he has been awarded a legal right. Legal rights are often conferred for moral reasons and moral rights may be affected by laws as by other circumstances, but the two are different. We will primarily focus on moral rights today.

A moral right is often thought of as anything upon which a moral argument can be based, but this is not the case. When we say that we should not torture animals for pleasure (or even perhaps for experimentation), we may mean to advance the claim that animals have a right not to be tortured or that people have a right to live in a society in which animal torture does not occur. But we may simply mean that it is wrong to torture animals, even if animals do not themselves possess rights and no other rights are violated. Of course we must always remember that whatever it is that we may mean we may still be mistaken. The point is that we will only find our errors by careful analysis of our own positons and the arguments against them. John Stuart Mill wrote of "duties of imperfect obligation" which are morally imperative although none of their beneficiaries is entitled to claim their performance as a right. He cited charity as an example of such an imperfect obligation. Perhaps kindness to animals is similar. (Mill: Utilitarianism--cited in Macklin, p.35)

Moral rights language is built upon tripartite claims of the form: X has a right to some thing T against Y, where X and Y are both persons (or at least entities) and T is a thing (material or immaterial) in dispute. Y is the person whose obligation corresponds to X's right, and who foots the bill for it. Sometimes Y is not specified and the speaker may be taking Y to mean any passerby or any or all members of some group or society at large, but we must be careful always to identify Y. The statement "George Collins has a right to health care," has very different implications if the Y who is to assure George's care is a specific doctor or the AMA or society at large.

Joel Feinberg (Feinberg, 1970) has described a different sense of rights in which Y is unspecified and cannot be identified. He calls these "manifesto rights" because they tend to appear in sweeping manifestos urging us to a higher moral plane. These generally mean not that I ought to grant Joe next door such rights but that all of us ought to work toward securing such rights for those who lack them. I think some of Feinberg's manifesto rights can be analyzed more clearly within our tripartite strucuture by allowing X and Y to represent groups as well as individuals. The rest seem to me to be not rights-claims at all but arguments that we should agree to create such rights by guaranteeing these things to those who lack them and need them.

Some kind of rights-claims imply that Y has a positive obligation to act or at least to be prepared to act to facilitate X's obtaining T. Some merely imply that Y should not interfere. Consider the difference between "I have a right to go to medical school because I am black, and so you should admit me," and "I have a right to go to medical school even if I am black, so don't file an interview report reflecting your prejudices." As we will see in the case of life and death decisions in the neonatal intensive care unit, the difference between rights implying obligations to act and rights implying obligations to refrain from interfering may be crucial to an analysis. Philosophers use many different terms to distinguish these types of rights, but perhaps strong rights and weak rights are as good as any.

Another distinction to be made is between absolute and non-absolute rights. There are very few absolutes in either morality or medicine and no great preponderance in their intersection. Most rights, whether to action or to non-interference, are what many philosophers call "prima facie" rights. Prima facie literally means "at first impression" and has come in ethics to mean valid but able to be over-ridden. As Feinberg has pointed out, it is really not rights that are prima facie but the claims or entitlements to which they give rise. In our discussion of informed consent, for instance, we will consider whether a depressed patient has a "right to know" about the risks of the electro-convulsive therapy being suggested to her. But such a right, if it exists, gives rise only to a prima facie claim to this knowledge, so we will then have to consider whether this claim may be overridden by her physician's obligation to refrain from giving her information that may harm her.

In analyzing a claim to rights language then, we must first determine whether the use of rights language is warranted, ascertaining whether each of the three parts of the rights-claim is present. That is, we must discover who has the supposed right, what it is a right to, and whom the right is against. We must distinguish between strong rights (rights to action) and weak rights (rights to non-interference) and between claims based on moral rights and claims based on legal rights. To evaluate the strength of the claim advanced based on this right, we must ascertain the origin of the right and its relative urgency or force as compared to other rights-claims that also apply to the situation in question.

The process sounds complex, but should not be difficult. Rights language is an important part of moral discourse today and one with which we should all become conversant so

that we can use it when it is called for and ignore it when
it is not. As well as an improved knowledge of the issues
listed on the program today, I hope that you will leave this
afternoon with additional practice in making the distinction.

REFERENCES

Editors   (1976).   Editors' note. Hastings Center Report
      6(5)33.
Englehard HT Jr (1979).   Rights to health care: a critical
      appraisal.   J Med Phil 4(2):113-117.
Heifetz MD, Mangel C (1975).   "The Right to Die." New York:
      GP Putnam's Sons.
In re appointment of a Guardian of the person of Maida Yetter.
      Docket No. 1973-533.   (PaCt. of Common Pleas, North-
      hampton Co. Orphan's Ct., June 6, 1973).
Macklin R (1976).   Moral concerns and appeals to rights.
      Hastings Center Report 6(5):31-32,34-38.

INTRODUCTION: THE RIGHT TO HEALTH CARE

Marc D. Basson

Director, CEHM
University of Michigan
Ann Arbor, Michigan

Stephen Stich approaches the question of the right to
health care from the point of view of an analytic philosopher.
He carefully dissects out the different sorts of claims that
might be implicit in an appeal to a right to health care.
He ends by arguing that the most controversial of these
claims, that of what he calls a moral right to health care,
is difficult indeed to argue for but that we do not need to
make such an argument, for a legal right can be established
even in the absence of a moral right. Stich suggests that
the creation of such a legal right would increase the general
quality of life and that this is a good motive for utilitarians
and non-utilitarians alike.

Stich ducks the question of exactly what sort of national
health insurance or care scheme he would have us establish,
noting that anything would be better than nothing. Congressman Pursell is more concerned with these practical considerations. He enumerates multiple instances of modern medical
technology which improve quality of care but also run up
quite a bill. Pursell urges that we consider cost-effectiveness and allocate our resources accordingly, for there is
only so much to go around.

While Stich urges the creation of a legal right to health
care even in the absence of an established moral right and
Pursell sounds a note of caution as to the possible extent
of such a right, others hesitate to create any such universal
right. "The idea of individual responsibility has been
submerged in individual rights -- rights or demands to be
guaranteed by beneficient Big Brother," writes John Knowles,

President of the Rockefeller Foundation. "One man's or woman's freedom in health is now another man's shackle in taxes and insurance premiums....The cost of individual irresponsibility in health has become prohibitive. The choice is in fact, over the long range, individual responsibility or social failure." (Quoted disapprovingly in Crawford, 1978)

Our case for this topic involves an inveterate alcoholic who refuses treatment for his life-threatening addiction and who demand palliation for its consequences. Such cases are common, according to those of Knowles's persuasion, and along with the cases of lung and cardiovascular disease in smokers and other preventable illnesses, constitute a strong argument against the creation of a uniform national right to health care. Leon Kass, for instance, suggests incorporating "inducements into the insurance plan by measures such as refusing or reducing benefits...to persons who continue to smoke." (Kass, 1975)

Some, such as Meredith Eiker whose work appears elsewhere in this volume, have urged the Veterans Administration Hospital system as a test case for extensive national health insurance or even socialized medicine. Others are struck by unfortunate cases such as this one in which the legally granted right to virtually unlimited health care backfires. The reader is referred to Kass (1975) and Crawford (1978) for an excellent introduction to this debate.

REFERENCES

Crawford, R (1978). You are dangerous to your health. Social Policy, Jan-Feb, 11-20.
Kass, L (1975). Regarding the end of medicine and the pursuit of health. Public Interest, 40(Summer): 11-42.

**Rights and Responsibilities in Modern Medicine: The Second
Volume in a Series on Ethics, Humanism, and Medicine: 11—13**
© 1981 Alan R. Liss, Inc., 150 Fifth Avenue, New York, NY 10011

THE RIGHT TO HEALTH CARE: WHAT IS IT AND WHAT
SHOULD WE DO ABOUT IT?

Case for Discussion

In 1930, a law was enacted guaranteeing American
veterans free health care and the Veterans Administration
Hospital system was established to provide this care. Under
the current law, veterans requiring care for service-
connected disabilities receive first priority while non-
service-connected disabilities receive second priority, but
this distinction is not made for patients ill enough to be
hospitalized. Because of the age and uniquely unlimited
guarantee of this system, many see it as a test case for the
right to health care in this country. The case described
below is not meant to depict the "typical" VA Hospital
admission, but it is by no means atypical either.

Gregory Collins is a 57-year-old World War II veteran
admitted to the Ann Arbor Veterans Administration Hospital
for the fourth time for alcoholic liver disease since he
moved to Michigan two years ago. He has signed out against
medical advice on two of these occasions.

Mr. Collins has been drinking up to two fifths of
whiskey per day for the last 15-20 years and smoked two packs
per day since he was fourteen. Other than multiple previous
hospitalizations for alcoholic liver disease, Mr. Collin's
past medical history is significant for three automobile
accidents (in 1963, 1966, and 1967) suffered while driving
intoxicated. The second of these left him without sight in
his left eye after the eye was pierced by a shard of glass.

He dropped out of school after eleventh grade and
worked on assembly lines and similar jobs until twelve years

ago when he was fired for absenteeism. He has been
unemployed since. He was married but his wife divorced him
because they "just didn't get along." He has one daughter,
now married, with whom he lives and who buys him his whiskey
with his Social Security.

This time Mr. Collins is brought to the hospital by
his son-in-law in a lethargic state and soon lapses into
hepatic coma, a condition in which the body's waste products
are no longer broken down by the malfunctioning liver and
thus accumulate and poison the brain. Most of the ward team
doubts he will servive.

After four days in an intensive care unit with one
attempt at peritoneal dialysis to cleanse his blood of wastes
and five more days of careful monitoring in a hospital ward,
he is finally returned to his baseline mental status. His
liver disease is irreversible, but the wastes can still be
metobolized slowly. His doctors tell him that if he abstains
from alcohol (as he has for nine days now), he can expect to
go on living. Otherwise, the next hospitalization for this
problem (which will certainly worsen if he continues to
drink) may well be his last.

Mr. Collins replies sorrowfully, "I guess I'm just a
terrible drunk. That's what I am, you know, a drunk. I just
can't quit, so I'll have to go on drinking and letting you
doctors fix me up just like you did this time until some day
when you can't and I am punished for my drinking." He is
offered referrals to Alcoholics Anonymous and a local therapy
group and refuses both. He is evaluated by a psychiatrist
who reports that there is no evidence that Mr. Collins really
wants to quit drinking and says Collins clearly understands
(at least intellectually) what he has been told.

The patient's daughter is contacted and it becomes
apparent from the conversation that she herself is a heavy
drinker and will not deprive the patient of his alcohol. She
insists that "a drink now and again never killed anyone. Why
don't you just find out what's wrong with him and fix it?"
despite all explanations. "After all," she adds, "the
government isn't paying you to give poor veterans lectures
about the way they live. You're supposed to cure them."

On the tenth hospital day, Mr. Collins signs out
against medical advice after a nurse refuses to bring him

some medicinal alcohol. His hospitalization cost the government (which pays for his care) over $4,000.

Is there a right to health care? Does Collins have
such a right? Should he? What limits, if any, should be
placed on such a right when it is created (as our government
has done for veterans)? What should be the proper goals of
such obligatory care and how far should it extend?

Rights and Responsibilities in Modern Medicine: The Second
Volume in a Series on Ethics, Humanism, and Medicine: 15–30
© 1981 Alan R. Liss, Inc.,150 Fifth Avenue, New York, NY 10011

THE MANY RIGHTS TO HEALTH AND HEALTH CARE

Stephen P. Stich

Department of Philosophy and Committee on the
History and Philosophy of Science
University of Maryland
College Park, MD   20742

I.   INTRODUCTION

When Mr. Basson, the Director of the Committee on Ethics,
Humanism and Medicine, asked me to participate in this conference, the topic he proposed was "the right to health care
or the right to health." I protested that this could cover
many different issues and asked for some clarification on
just what he wanted me to talk about. The response was an
embarrassed silence, followed by some mumbled muttering
about deciding for myself what the proposed topic might mean.
Now those of you who know Mr. Basson are well aware that he
is not a man given to mumbling, nor is he easily embarrassed.
I take this uncharacteristic behavior to be a symptom that
many physicians and medical students, even philosophically
sophisticated ones like Mr. Basson, are perplexed about what
a right to health or health care might be. Some of this
perplexity, as we shall see, may be traced to genuinely
vexing ethical quandries. However, a good deal of the puz-
zlement is rooted in careless thinking and the failure to
keep in mind some relatively straightforward distinctions.
Since distinctions are the philosopher's stock in trade, I
will devote much of my time in this lecture to drawing a few
that are crucial if we are to think clearly about rights to
health and health care. My central theme will be that there
are many quite distinct claims one might be making in
asserting a right to health or a right to health care. Some
of these claims are important, some banal; some raise profound moral issues, while others are trivially true or
trivially false. My second theme, which will make its
appearance toward the end of the lecture, is that the various

questions we will distinguish, while surely interconnected, are not so tightly bound to one another as has sometimes been imagined. In particular, I will urge that a case can be made for a legal right to health care which does not pre-suppose a moral right.

II. SOME DISTINCTIONS

The notion of a right is so central to our moral and social "forms of life" that it resists easy definition. This has not, however, prevented a small army of philosophers, lawyers and others from trying their hands at producing just such a definition.[1] And I must confess a certain temptation to use this conference as an excuse to join their ranks and produce a definition of my own. But in the interest of brevity I will forbear. Instead I will assume that we all have a rough but workable intuitive grasp of what a right is, and I will devote my efforts to limning some sub-categories under the larger heading of rights.

A. Legal Rights and Moral Rights

Some rights are spelled out quite explicitly in the Constitution or in various pieces of legislation. These are the paradigm cases of *legal rights*, rights which have the force of law. Not all legal rights are explicitly specified in written law, however. In many countries there are also common law legal rights that have never been articulated in a constitution or in legislation. In addition there are many legal rights that the courts have found to be "implicit" in the Constitution or in various pieces of legislation, though they are hardly manifest in the written word. The right to use a contraceptive and the right to have an abortion are a pair of relatively recent - and controversial - addi-tions to this category of implicit constitutional rights.

Moral rights, in contrast to legal rights, are those which a person has not in virtue of any law, but merely in virtue of being a person in the particular situation he or she may be in. They are, if you will, rights sanctioned by the moral law, not by any legislative code. Most of us hold

1. For a particularly sophisticated attempt, cf. Feinberg (1970).

moral views which accord people a significant range of rights quite independently of whether these rights are sanctioned by law. The right to speak one's mind, to practice the religion of one's choice (or none at all), and the right to a fair trial are a few relatively uncontroversial examples.

The relation between legal rights and moral rights is a complicated matter that will loom large later in my talk. For the moment, however, let me make a few obvious observations about that complex relation. First, it is clear that legal rights and moral rights do not necessarily coincide. There are legal rights which do not simply sanction pre-existing moral rights, and there are moral rights which are not sanctioned by the law. A single historical example will serve to illustrate both phenomena. In the years prior to the Emancipation Proclamation an American slave owner had a clear legal right to recapture a runaway slave, even in a free state. But though a slave owner in those years had a *legal* right to recapture "his" runaway slave, many people at the time denied that he had any *moral* right to do so, a view which I would hope is shared by everyone in this audience. On the other hand, all of us and many of our pre-Civil War forebearers believe that a runaway slave, indeed any slave, had a moral right to be free. But the right not to spend the remainder of his days in bondage was not, in those years, a legal right. So moral rights and legal rights can and do diverge. Nor, and this is my second point, is it always lamentable when they do diverge. Let me use two other examples to make the point. I am inclined to think that parents usually have a right to respect and solicitude from their grown children. Also, I would argue that if a professor tells his class that 50% of their course grades will be determined by the final exam, then each student has a right to a grade which is so determined. In both cases the rights in question are moral rights, not legal rights. And I think most of us would agree that these moral rights are best *not* given the sanction of law.

B. Action Rights and Recipient Rights

What I shall call an "action right" is a right to do something, if I choose to and if I can, without being interfered with. The idea of an *action* or of *doing* something must be construed broadly to include actions in which one doesn't do much of anything - remaining silent, for example. It must also include being or remaining in various states of body or mind - as in the right to go unwashed or to believe that God is dead.

It is important to stress that action rights are rights to do something without interference, *if one can*. One of the "percs" of my job is the right to use the university's running track. I may jog as long and as often as I wish. But if the truth be known I have never succeeded in running more than about ten miles, and on that occasion my knees made me aware of the folly of my deed in no uncertain terms. The lamentable fact is that I *cannot* run marathon distances. But it would be a bad joke if I were to protest that my right to run at the university track had been impinged because I could not run twenty six miles. All of this is clear enough. However, there are other cases where matters are murkier, where the line between inability and interference is hard to locate. Suppose, for example, that the university regularly locks the fence surrounding the track. Are they still respecting my right to unlimited use of the facility? Let us suppose that if I succeeded in scaling the fence the campus police would not interfere and would have no objection to my using the track. Does the locked fence nonetheless count as an interference with my right to use the track? Does the answer perhaps turn on how high the fence is? The issue is a frivolous one of course, but it illustrates a serious point. The way in which we draw the line between inability and interference will often determine whether a right has been respected or violated. Thus our views on how to locate this boundary will sometimes have profound moral implications. Consider, for example, the right of handicapped citizens to use public facilities. Is this right violated if the facilities are not readily accessible to persons in wheelchairs? How we answer will depend largely on whether we view this as a case of inability or as a case of interference.

Action rights are sometimes called "negative rights" or "liberties." And, indeed, many of our traditional liberties fall into this category. The right to practice whatever religion I choose is an action right, as is the right to print and offer for sale anything, or almost anything, I wish. Both of these are legal rights, and many would argue that they are moral rights as well. Another example of an action right is the right, claimed by gay liberation advocates, to engage in private sexual acts with a consenting adult partner of the same sex. Supporters of gay liberation contend that this is a moral right and *ought* also to be a legal right, though in many places it is not.

What I shall call "recipient rights" are rights to receive some object or service from another person, from an organization, or from the government. A recipient right is not adequately specified unless the person or institution who is obliged to provide the good or service has been indicated. So long as I continue to reside in Prince George's County, Maryland, for example, my children have a right to an elementary and secondary school education, *provided by the county*. And if I should die before they are grown, they have a right to certain payments *from the Social Security Administration*. But they would have no right to any payments from the county, nor do they have any right to an elementary school education provided by the Social Security Administration. Since recipient rights are rights to receive something from a specified provider, they generally impose special obligations on those who must do the providing. Action rights, by contrast, commonly impose on all of us the "negative" obligation to refrain from interfering with the protected action. Matters are not quite so tidy as this suggests, however, since certain action rights impose the obligation of non-interference only on a specific group or institution - most often the government. My right to worship as I please imposes an obligation on the State of Maryland not to penalize me should I adopt an unconventional religion. To do so would be to violate my legal right of free worship. But if my father cuts me out of his will because of my new religion, he has not violated this right. The right imposes no obligation on him.

From time to time in the debate on the right to health care one finds the startling argument that there could not be a right to health care since the notion of a recipient right is somehow confused and contradictory. The only real rights, it is said, are action rights or liberties.[2] But

2. Consider, for example, the following passage from Szasz (1969): "In the sense specified above,... there can be no such thing as a right to treatment. Conceiving of a person's body as his possession - like his automobile or watch (though no doubt more valuable) - it is just as nonsensical to speak of his right to have his body repaired as it would be to speak of his right to have his automobile or watch repaired." (477) But surely it is not in the least nonsensical to

this last claim is about as wrong headed as a claim can be.
After all, contract rights are paradigm cases of recipient
rights, and surely there is nothing confused or contradictory
about the notion of a contract right. Indeed, as a member
of a pre-paid health maintenance organization I have a contract right to health care, provided by the organization.
So there is one reading of the question, "Is there a right
to health care?" to which the answer is, trivially *yes*.

Though the distinction between action and recipient
rights is generally pretty clear, there are some cases that
resist ready classification. Many of these cases arise when
the "good or service" to which one has a right might plausibly be viewed also as a liberty. Consider an example. Some
years ago (perhaps still) lounge chairs were set out on
sunny days in the Jardin de Luxembourg in Paris. To sit in
one, it was necessary to buy a ticket for a small sum from
an old man in uniform who ambled around the park. (I was
told that the right to sell tickets was accorded to elderly
war veterans as a means of supplementing their incomes,
though I am not sure this is correct.) Having bought a
ticket one had a right to sun oneself in a lounge chair for
the rest of the day. Was this an action right - a right to
do something - or a recipient right? The answer is not
entirely clear; it seems to be an intermediate case.

C. Health and Health Care

The last distinction on my list is the obvious distinction between health and health care. Oddly enough, the
distinction itself is clearer than the notions being distinguished. Health is a state (or perhaps a combination of
states) while health care is a sort of service (or perhaps
many sorts). And while there is abundant room for dispute
over what states count as healthy and what services count as
health care services, there is no temptation to count any

-----

speak of a right to have one's automobile repaired. The
warrantees that come with new cars give the buyer the right
to have his car repaired at the manufacturer's expense for
a stipulated length of time. For two other versions of the
curious view that the idea of a recipient right is somehow
muddled, cf. the quotes from Sade (1974) and Kuenzi (1973)
given in Beauchamp and Faden (1979).

service as a part of health, nor any state as a part of
health care. Some examples may clarify the point. Are old
age, extreme ugliness or homosexuality unhealthy, and their
opposites, youth, beauty and heterosexuality, a part of good
health? The answers are far from clear. But whatever we
decide about the relation between beauty and health, it is
clear that beauty is no part of health *care*. To suggest
that it is would be to commit what it was once fashionable
to call a "category mistake." On the other side, consider
cosmetic surgery, psychoanalysis or laetrile therapy. Do
any of these count as health care? Once again there is ample
room for dispute, though to consider any of these as a part
of health would be to commit a "logical howler."

III. RIGHTS TO HEALTH AND HEALTH CARE: SOME INTERPRETATIONS

The three distinctions we have drawn above generate a
total of eight possible readings that might be assigned to
the question: *Is there a right to health or health care?*
We might be asking about a moral action right to health, a
legal recipient right to health care, etc. The possibilities
are systematically displayed in figure 1. Actually, figure 1

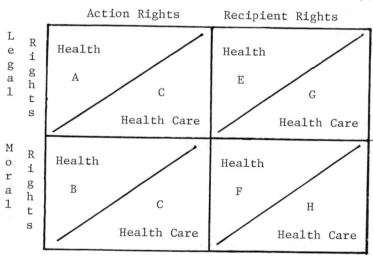

Figure 1

does not exhaust the possibilities we have elaborated, because recipient rights are not fully specified unless we

specify the provider. Thus category G would contain both the legal right to health care from a health maintenance organization (which I have), and the legal right to health care from the government (which I do not have). Keeping this in mind, let me run through the chart and comment brief-ly on each of the categories.

Categories A and B

An action right to health would be a right not to have one's health interfered with. It would oblige others to refrain from environmental polution, dangerous action in the presence of others, etc. There is no broad legal right to health, though there are many specific laws controlling or prohibiting actions that are harmful to the health of others. But what about category B? Is there a moral action right to health? Before taking a stand on that issue we would do well to reflect on how broad a conception of health we have in mind. If we are to count people as unhealthy only when they are seriously ill or injured, then there is considerable plausibility to the claim that we have a moral action right to health - a right to insist that others not engage in actions that will injure us or make us ill. But if such conditions as anxiety are to count as making us unhealthy, then the case for a moral right to health is much less con-vincing. A good number of the President's recent foreign policy decisions have substantially increased my level of anxiety. But I would be reluctant to claim that the Presi-dent has thereby violated my rights.

A particularly vexing issue that arises in connection with an action right to health is the role probabilities should play in our deliberations about rights. If there is a substance that always causes cancer when inhaled, and if my neighbor insists in spraying his roses with the stuff while I am down wind of him, I have a right to insist that he stop. But suppose there is a substance which has some relatively modest probability of causing cancer. Have I a right to insist it not be released into the atmosphere any-where near me? The case is hardly a hypothetical one, since tobacco smoke is just such a substance.

This is an appropriate place to raise a general question about rights. Suppose it is agreed that I have a certain right, and that the right has been violated. What follows?

What redress is appropriate from the person or institution responsible for violating my rights? The answer can only be *it depends*. If the right in question is a legal right, then the law itself will sometimes specify the sort of redress that is appropriate. Sometimes, however, the law will remain silent on the issue. When the right in question is a moral right, the issue of appropriate redress is often a vexing one. It is quite possible for a pair of sensible observers to agree that a moral right has been violated, while disagreeing quite markedly on what should be done about it. For the issue of redress is a second, and often largely separate, moral question. The matter is relevant to our current concerns since there are many who argue that when a moral action right to health care has been violated, the victim acquires a recipient right to appropriate health care treatment, to be provided either by the person who has violated his rights or by the government.[3] This is not an unreasonable view, and I am prepared to be convinced that it is the right one. But my present point is that some convincing - some additional moral argument - is necessary. It is not a conceptual truth, a mere tautology, that a person whose right to health has been violated ought to be compensated with appropriate health care.

Categories C and D

An action right to health care would be a right to receive health care if one chooses and if one can, without interference. One might think that there is a clear moral right here as well as a clear legal right. If I choose to receive a certain treatment from my doctor, and if I can receive it from her, others should not interfere. Unfortunately, however, what looks at first to be an obvious platitude turns out to mask a number of moral controversies. Consider first the question of what counts as interference. If the treatment in question is to be administered in a certain hospital and you forceably prevent me from entering the hospital, then surely you have violated my right to health care (not to speak of a number of other rights). But suppose that my entry is barred not for capricious reasons, but for a malicious one. Suppose, for example, that I am black and no blacks are allowed to enter the hospital. Is my right to health care violated in this case? Or suppose,

3.   Cf. Beauchamp and Faden (1979), p. 124.

rather, that I am simply poor, and the hospital will permit no one to use its facilities without a reasonable guarantee that it will be paid. Does *this* count as a violation of my action right to health care? The problem, of course, is simply a particular instance of a more general problem raised earlier: How shall we draw the boundary between interference and inability? If we draw that boundary so as to include the case of the poor patient under the heading of interference, then an action right to health care will entail a recipient right as well.

Quite a different issue concerning action rights to health care arises when we attend more carefully to just what counts as *health* care. If laetrile "therapy" is to be included under the heading of health care, then there are many places where the legal action right to health care is restricted. For, in those places, I cannot be treated with laetrile even though I want to and my doctor is willing to treat me. Many of those who are unhappy with this state of affairs assert that there is a moral action right in these cases, and that the law ought to recognize this moral right. Cases of a slightly different sort arise when an uncontroversial therapy is provided by a controversial therapist. There are no qualms, moral or legal, if my doctor prescribes penicillin for my strep throat. But if the same course of treatment is prescribed by my plumber, the law respects no action right for me to receive the treatment. Some, like Thomas Szasz, see this legal restriction as an infringement on the moral action right to health care.[4]

Categories E Through H

Let us turn now to the second column in our chart, the one headed "recipient rights." Here, it would seem, two of our four categories can be dismissed quickly. Categories E and F are, respectively, legal and moral recipient rights to health. But, as we noted earlier, there can be no recipient right to a good or service unless there is some person or institution who is obligated to provide the good or service. And it is an axiom of moral philosophy that one cannot be obligated to do something one cannot do. But providing health looks to be a paradigm case of what persons and institutions cannot do. Health care can be provided;

4. See, for example, Szasz (1975).

health, alas, cannot. So it looks like there simply cannot
be a recipient right to health, be it legal or moral. There
is, of course, no analogous problem about recipient rights
to health care. We have already noted that certain people
have legal rights to health care: I have a right to health
care provided by my health maintenance organization; all
residents of the United Kingdom have a right to health care
provided by the National Health Service. However, many
people in this country have no legal right to health care.

Of the many issues that have been catalogued in this
talk, the most topical and the most hotly debated is whether
there *should* be some sort of general legal right to health
care provided by the government. Much of the debate in this
area, on both sides of the issue, appears to take it for
granted that to resolve the question we must establish whether
or not there is a *moral* right to government provided health
care. The assumption seems to be that the only plausible
justification for establishing a legal right is the existence
of an antecedent moral right - that justification for a category G right must flow from a category H right. It is understandable enough that the parties to the dispute should make
this assumption, for there is a conspicuous and venerable
precedent here. Many of the most important historical arguments over the establishment of a legal right have turned on
making the case for a moral right. This was the structure
of the principal argument against slavery: slaves have a
moral right to liberty, and thus they should have the legal
right as well. In more recent times the same pattern of
argument has been used with great success by the civil rights
movement: black people have a moral right to vote, to use
public facilities, etc., and thus we should enact a parallel
legal right. Much the same form of argument is used by gay
rights advocates, feminists, animal liberation advocates and
others. In most of these cases the right being advocated is
an action right rather than a recipient right, and thus the
parallel with a recipient right to health care is not a perfect one. Nonetheless, the salience in our civic lives of
arguments from moral rights to legal rights makes it quite
unsurprising that many assume this is the only way in which
a legal right can sensibly be justified. However, though
the assumption is a pervasive one, I am convinced that it is
wrong. More specifically, I hold that demonstrating the
existence of an antecedent moral right is neither the only
way, nor necessarily the best way, to argue for enactment
of a legal recipient right. This is the theme that will

occupy me for the remainder of my talk.

Before taking up the theme, however, let me note one
reason to *hope* I am right. Very simply, the reason is this.
If I am wrong, and if we must wait for a convincing demonstration or refutation of the moral right to health care
before deciding whether we should have a legal right, then
I fear we may have a very long wait indeed. To show that
there is a moral right to health care would, presumably,
require showing how this right followed from a more general
moral theory. But it is no easy matter to derive recipient
right claims from general moral theories. And, as Norman
Daniels has recently shown, the derivability of a recipient
right to health care even from the most sympathetic general
theory is an open question which is not likely to be soon
settled.[5] But if I am right, we can do an end run around
these difficulties, and make a case for a legal right which
is quite independent of the parallel moral right.

IV. LEGAL RIGHTS WITHOUT MORAL RIGHTS

Come to think of it, most of us must think there is a
way to justify legal recipient rights without resting them
on moral rights. Deriving moral recipient rights from
general moral theories is, as we have noted, generally a
tricky business. Yet we have lots of legal recipient rights,
and with an occasional caveat most of us think that we *should*
have these rights, even though we have no idea how to derive
the parallel moral right from a moral theory. So we must
think there is some other sort of reason why we should have
these legal rights, a reason that does not turn on moral
rights at all. What could this reason be? Let us consider
a thoroughly mundane example.

As a resident of the town of University Park, Maryland,
I have a right to have my garbage collected by the town. In
terms of the taxonomy we have developed, this is a legal
recipient right. I am convinced that there ought to be such
a legal right in my community, and it is clear that the

5. Cf. Daniels (1979). Daniels' paper is the most philosophically sophisticated essay I know of on the topic of the
right to health care. Though he too seems to share the wide-
spread assumption that a legal right to health care must be
justified by an appeal to an antecedent moral right.

overwhelming majority of my neighbors agree. If a town councilman were to propose abolishing the right, no one would take him seriously. But now why do my neighbors and I think that we should have a legal right to have our trash collected by the town. Is it because we think there is a moral right to trash collection? Surely not. Rather, we think we should retain our legal right to trash collection because we think our community is a *better* one with such a right in place than without. If we did not have trash collection provided by the town, the neighborhood would be less tidy, less attractive and less healthy. The need to arrange for private trash collection would impose a distressing financial burden on the poorer residents of the community, and it would be an unwelcome nuisance for the rest of us. In short, the *quality of life* in the community would be diminished if our right to trash collection were revoked.

Now it is my contention that this concern with the quality of community life underlies a good number of our legal recipient rights. We think we *ought* to have rights to trash collection, snow removal, water and sewer hook-ups, emergency ambulance service, insect control programs, and many others, not because we think there is a moral right to have these services provided by the government, but because having these legal rights improves the quality of life in our society.

At this point some of you, no doubt, will be itching to ask just exactly what I mean by the quality of life. But your itches will have to remain unscratched, for I do not propose to provide a theory detailing the constituents of the quality of life and how they shall be measured. Nor is my refusal rooted in mere perversity. Rather, I am struck by the fact that the defense of legal recipient rights that I am proposing is compatible with a range of quite different views on what constitutes the quality of life. If you are a utilitarian, then you will take the quality of an individual life to be a function of the amount of pleasure or happiness in that life; and you will take the measure of the quality of life in a community to be the arithmetic mean of the quality of individual lives. So for the utilitarian, the right to trash collection ought to be retained because doing so will lead to more happiness, on the average, than revoking the right. But perhaps you are not a utilitarian. Perhaps you would include more than happiness in assessing the quality of a life; or perhaps you would urge that the quality of life in a community is not simply the mean of the quality of individual lives. If this is the case, then I invite you to reckon the quality of life as you will. It is my conjecture that for almost all of us, despite the diversity in the ways it is reckoned, the quality of community life comes out higher with public trash collection than without.

There is yet another way in which you could disagree with a utilitarian. The utilitarian contends that what we ought to do is what maximizes the average quality of life. So for the utilitarian, if the quality of life is higher with public trash collection than without, it follows straightway that we ought to have it. But perhaps you do not think that we ought *always* to do what will maximize the quality of life. You think that other considerations must play a role in deciding what ought to be done. But if you hold such a view, the "quality of life argument" for recipient rights may still often sway you. For it is unlikely that you think the quality of life is irrelevant in deciding what ought to be done. Rather, you think that other considerations can sometimes override a concern with the quality of life. But, in the trash collection case at least, few of us have principled concerns that would override the quality of life argument. It is my suspicion that the robustness of public support for trash collection and certain other recipient rights can be traced to the fact that a quality of life argument for these rights is insensitive to quite substantial variations in the way we assess the quality of life and in the factors that we take to override concern with the quality of life.

Let us return, finally, to the question of health care. Should there be a legal recipient right to health care provided or paid for by the government? I am strongly inclined to think that the answer is yes. The reason I would offer has nothing to do with a moral right to health care. Rather, it is my conviction that a national health insurance scheme would substantially improve the quality of life in our nation. It would reduce very substantially the suffering now endured by those in our society who cannot afford the medical care they need; it would quiet the anxiety that many of us feel about the financial consequences of catastrophic illness in our families; and it would be a substantial step in reducing those social inequalities that arise not because of unequal merit, but because of racial discrimination and accidents of birth. The experience of those who have lived in societies with national health plans - as I have in Britain - is instructive here. Though there is generally some grousing and political controversy about the quantity and quality of service provided, there is almost no serious opposition to retaining the system as a whole. The quality of life with a national health service is unmistakably higher than it would be without.

There remains one fundamentally important question that I have so far tucked under the rug. Before closing, let me at least point to the ugly bump it makes. I have argued that a legal recipient right to health care provided by the government - a national health insurance scheme - *ought* to be enacted, because the quality of life in our society would improve with enactment of such a scheme. What I have tucked under the rug is the fact that there are many different sorts of national health insurance plans, and they differ on many dimensions. Here the analogy with trash collection breaks down. Trash collection plans vary considerably less than national health insurance plans. Once it is agreed that *some* national health insurance scheme ought to be enacted, we must go on to decide *how much* health care it ought to provide. Possible answers range from the "decent minimum" urged by Fried,[6] through the broad range of services provided by Britain's National Health Service, to plans that would offer face lifts to middle aged matrons, and psychoanalysis to intellectuals suffering from Weltschmertz. Obviously, the more generous the benefits, the more costly the plan would be. If we ought to adopt one such plan, which one should it be? I must confess that this is a question for which I have no fully satisfactory answer. But I am convinced that almost any choice along the continuum between Fried's decent minimum and Britain's National Health Service would mark a substantial improvement in the quality of our lives and the decency of our society. If I have convinced you of this much, I will be well satisfied.

REFERENCES

Beauchamp TL, Faden RR (1979). The right to health and the right to health care. J of Medicine and Philosophy 4,2.
Daniels N (1979). Rights to health care and distributive justice: programmatic worries. J of Medicine and Philosophy 4,2.
Feinberg J (1970). The nature and value of rights. J of Value Inquiry, 4,4. Reprinted in Gorovitz et al (1976).

6. Cf. Fried (1976).

Fried C (1976). Equality and rights in medical care. Hastings Center Report, 6,1.

Gorovitz S, Jameton AL, Macklin R, O'Connor JM, Perrin EV, St. Clair BP, Sherwin S (eds) (1976). "Moral Problems in Medicine." Englewood Cliffs, NJ: Prentice-Hall.

Kuenzi DE (1973). Health care, a right? Missouri Medicine, 70,1.

Sade R (1974). Is health care a right? Image 7,1.

Szasz T (1969). The right to health. Georgetown Law Journal 57. Reprinted in Gorovitz et al (1976). Page reference in text is to this version.

Szasz T (1975). "Ceremonial Chemistry." Garden City, NY: Anchor Books.

Rights and Responsibilities in Modern Medicine: The Second
Volume in a Series on Ethics, Humanism, and Medicine: 31—39
© 1981 Alan R. Liss, Inc., 150 Fifth Avenue, New York, NY 10011

RIGHT TO HEALTH CARE:
WHAT IS IT AND WHAT SHOULD WE DO ABOUT IT?

Congressman Carl D. Pursell
United States House of Representatives
Washington, D.C.

No one disputes the right to some health care
for every citizen in the United States. But
concerns have been expressed by many people
about the availability of these health care
services, and the quality and cost of such services
as well as the lack of emphasis upon the prevention of diseases.

How much health care should be provided to
each individual citizen? Medical practice is
based upon the theory that one should do everything possible for the individual patient, but
who looks at the marginal gains to each individual
versus the threats to the welfare of the whole from
the continually escalating costs. Public responsibility has been assumed for financing health care
for certain groups: those include the indigent
sick, (through Medicaid, which is left to individual
states for implementation), and the elderly (through
Medicare, which is part of the federal Social
Security system), the mentally ill, members of the
armed forces and veterans, and indigent American
Indians and migrant workers. Despite all this,
health care still remains largely dependent upon
the private system with 30% of the expenditures
for total health care coming from private sources
in 1977.

"In 1978 the nation's health bill was 183
billion dollars. Over 40% of this amount went
towards hospital bills. The average hospital stay
now costs $1,300. This is up 1000% since 1959

compared to a 236% increase in consumer prices
as a whole. In 1978 more than 38 billion dollars
was spent on Medicaid and Medicare, far exceeding
the original estimate when these public health
programs were enacted over a decade ago.

"There are a number of reasons for our escalating
health care costs, including: overall inflation,
the cost of complying with governmental regulations,
the growth of our elderly population coupled with
expanded health care benefits and increased demand
for services, malpractice awards and related
factors such as overprescribing and overtesting,
and, finally, heavy investment in new technology."[1]

It has been estimated that health care costs
are rising 1 million dollars per hour, 24 hours
a day, doubling every five years.[2] These rising
health care costs mean significantly higher amounts
of resources are diverted from other sectors and/or
taxes must be increased to meet the high outlay
from federal health programs. Individuals must
pay higher premiums for health insurance and thus
have less money available for other goods and
services. While we can all generally agree with
the concept of the need to curb the spiralling
costs of health care, we find ourselves confronted
with ethical decisions concerning how much to pay
for health care services. How much is any individual
human life worth? Ought we not to try to do
everything possible to offer a therapeutic course of
treatment for each individual in need of care in
order to attempt to restore them to good health?
These are ethical questions that get at the heart
of your conference today. As a legislator faced
with the decisions that relate to health and
social welfare through my work as a committee
member on the Labor/HEW Appropriations Subcommittee,
I am aware of the need to face these issues. I
applaud your efforts to integrate the study of
such ethical and moral issues within your educational
program.

Technological advances are important to the
health and welfare of our individual citizens. Who
would deny the life-saving services such as coronary
bypass surgery and electronic fetal monitoring?
Costs for coronary bypass surgery generally average
$10,000 or more per case, Electronic monitoring is

now used in over half the obstetrical cases
at a yearly direct cost of over $80 million
dollars. Who is and who should consider the cost
benefits of such programs? Should the federal
government attempt to regulate the expenditures
for health care or should individual health care
workers be made more cognizant of the costs of
their decisions?

If the artificial pancreas now being investi-
gated were shown to be potentially useful to the
extimated 4 million Americans with diabetes, what
fraction of our resources should be given to this
and at what costs to others dependent on the
common pool of federal funds? If an effective
artificial heart were found, who should be
considered for replacement-all individuals with
heart proglems or just selected persons? If
only selected individuals then who will determine
the criteria for replacement therapy and what will
these criteria be? Of equal importance is who
should finance these costly health services?

Ten percent of the population still has no
provision for financing their health care through
third party payments. Catastrophic costs of
extended hospital illness is another area of
concern for many individuals. What should be the
role of both state and federal government in
regulating these health care services?

It is a well known fact that persons over 65
represent a growing proportion of our population.
Currently they represent 11% of the total population, yet they constitute 25% of all hospital
admissions and utilize 38% of all impatient
days of care. The per-capita expenditures for
the aged are about 3.5 times greater than for
younger people due to the complexity and chronicity
of health problems found in the elderly.

Personal expenditure in the U.S. for medical
care has risen dramatically. Over 1 billion a
year is now spent on patent medicine, much of
which is worthless, some of which are even harmful.
With adequate education related to individual
health needs many of these funds could be redirected
to more useful expenditures for health care.
Who is responsible for designing a health education
program for our citizens? Which of the many health

professional groups will assume primary responsibility for health education and prevention of diseases?

In 1971 the U.S. was spending 77 billion for health care or roughly 6% of the Gross National Product. Latest estimates for 1979 indicate that total expenditures will be over 200 billion which is over 9% of the G.N.P. This is an increase of over 125 billion in just 8 years! At that rate in five years we will be spending 300 billion. Yet despite spending more money per-capita on health care than any other nation on earth, the U.S. is lagging well behind other countries in infant mortality and in other indices of health. In fact, the U.S. has fallen from 6th place among nations with the lowest infant mortality rates in 1959 to 16th place in 1971. The chances of dying from cancer have not changed significantly in the last 35 years. Despite a recent budget of 800 million for the National Cancer Institute, which was just increased to one billion this year, cancer remains the second leading cause of death, accounting for about 17% of all deaths in America. Greater attention must be focused on environmental causes and greater attention given to prevention of environmental pollutants if the battle against cancer is to be won. Although accidents are the leading cause of death for Americans between the age of one and 38 the management of medical emergencies is one of the weakest segments of the health care delivery system in the U.S.

While there is one doctor for every 645 people, there is only one general or primary care physician for every 4,771 persons. Specialization of physicians has resulted in serious imbalances in the geographic distribution of physician's services. A renewed interest in family practice has recently developed due to recognition of the problems of access and the high cost of specialized care.

Of the ten priorities addressed in the National Health Planning and Resource Development Act of 1974 (Public Law 93-641) the top priority was the need to provide primary health care to underserved areas. Congress has authorized many programs to meet this purpose, such as community health

centers, migrant and Indian health programs, mental
health centers and the National Health Service Corp.

Placing physicians in shortage areas and charging
prevailing rates for services may have little impact
if the major deterrent to appropriate utilization
of primary health services are poverty, lack of
transportation and fear or distrust of health
professionals who are alien to the culture of the
area. The greater incidence of health problems are
because of limited health resources, transportation
barriers, high rates of poverty, limited education
and cultural attitudes which create barriers between
residents of an area and health professionals.

Comprehensive Health Centers established by
HEW are one approach to attempt to meet the needs
of underserved communities. These Centers provide
primary medical, dental, and nutritional programs,
transportation services, environmental health
services, home health care and child development
programs. As yet few in number the Comprehensive
Health Center concept does demonstrate the effective
use of a broad system approach to meeting health
care needs.

Central cities and rural areas are characterized
by high rates of poverty and limited education.
Rural populations tend to be skewed toward a high
concentration of children, while both central city
and rural areas have a disproportionate share of
aged persons. Health problems vary in severity
and kind according to the geographical area,
with high blood pressure, diabetes, urinary tract
infections, anemia, TB, intestinal disorders, eye
and skin disease frequently found in adults in
rural America. Many rural children in poverty
areas suffer from chronic skin infections as well
as rickets, intestinal parasites and chronic infection
of the ears, with resulting partial deafness. A
1975 survey of the Rio Grande valley of Texas
indicated high infant mortality and the prevelance
of such preventable diseases as whooping cough,
tuberculosis, and typhus. Infant mortality rates
tend to be especially high in underserved areas.
For example, in 1974 the infant mortality rate
in South Carolina was 64% above the national
average. Deaths of infants in the first 28 days
after birth were 70% above the national average

in the District of Columbia.

Another priority in health planning and
resource development is the utilization of nurse
clinicians and physician's assistants in the delivery
of much needed primary care services. The Health
Professional Assistant Act of 1976 has provided
for a federal effort to support training programs
for the education of such practitioners, in the
hopes of providing care to underserved areas.

The massive expenditures for health care and
the intensive emphasis upon care serve to highlight
the lack of emphasis on the detection and prevention
of disease. Health education, rehabilitation
services and lower cost chronic care including
nursing home facilities have all been slighted.
We have emphasized high cost hospital based
technologies to the neglect of other services
where the benefits can be much greater relative to
the costs incurred. For example, legislation for
coverage of costs of renal dialysis was passed
long before legislation was enacted to stimulate
the detection and treatment of hypertension,
yet many more people are affected by high blood
pressure than by kidney failure.

Health insurance too has generally emphasized
hospital and surgical expenses. Coverage is far
less extensive for regular medical care, dental
care, drugs, and home health services. As of
1975 about 90% of hospital care expense was paid
by 3rd party payers, of this 37% was by private
health insurance, and 53% by the government. 63%
of the payments to physicians comes from 3rd party
coverage while only 14% of drug and dental expenses
are covered by insurance of any kind.[3] Alternative
programs such as hospices, home care, and day care
may prove less costly and more suitable for some
people than hospital care services, yet these
programs are frequently not covered. Should not
third party reimbursement allow for the choice
of the most effective plan of care in terms of
cost and suitability to both patient and families?

Prehospital rescue units contribute to
increased survival of patients with cardiac
arrest. Reasonable decision making would be to
ascertain the cost per life saved and determine
if a universal program of implementation is worthy

of consideration. Two critical questions must be
answered. What can really be achieved? Are the
benefits of wide application such as to warrant
displacing something else? Unfortunately, this has
not been done. Most communities are now trying to
implement such pre-hospital programs through voluntary support by citizens of the community. While
this service is undoubtedly useful one has to
wonder why we cannot raise money to put toward
health education in order to prevent such costly
health disasters.

Ethical dilemmas come into focus sharply when
we attempt to set a monetary value on human life.
Perhaps the dilemma is unnecessarily intensified
by the wide-spread misconception that the principal
objective of medical practice is prevention of
death. Only a small fraction of surgery and
non-surgery encounters involve life and death
decisions; most are directed at relief of physical
or emotional discomfort or disability. How much
are we willing to pay for the attempted relief of
these symptoms?

There are a number of medical procedures
which were at one time practiced widely in this
country and are now virtually abandoned because
they were ultimately found to be of little value.
For example, internal mammary artery ligation for
coronary artery disease. Although tonsillectomy
has an important place in medical practice some
pediatricians suggest that over 90% of the 1
million children who undergo tonsillectomies yearly
do so unnecessarily. The 444 million in expenditures
for T & A's could have been reduced to 40 million
dollars, the number of hospital days reduced
proportionately and the number of deaths from
general anesthesia might be cut from 70 to 7,
if unnecessary T & A's were not done. Use of
respiratory therapy has increased in recent years,
yet concern is voiced of the harm to patients
from possible excessive use. Who is to assume
the responsibility for monitoring these activities;
the health professionals, the consumer or the
government?

The volume of legislation relevant to health
care has grown impressively in this decade. As
a consequence of various congressional hearings the

federal government is now significantly interested and
involved in bioethical questions in addition to their interest
in medical economics and the health delivery problems. Disease
prevention, nutrition and the environment have all been
public health and Congressional concerns for many years. We
recognize that most money spent on a personal health care
system is mainly oriented to treating existing illness, yet
it is recognized that future improvements in the level of
health in Americans may lie mainly in the improvement of the
environment, moderating self imposed risks and moderating
our style of living. For example: the annual carnage on
our highways generates costly demands on the health care system,
but the behavior of the individual and the condition of the
car depends upon social, cultural and economic factors.
Also, evidence is mounting that the kinds of food and liquor
we consume in our generally affluent, sendentary society
are major factors associated with cancer, cardiovascular
disease and other chronic disabilities.

Prevention should become the paramount element in medical
care with health maintenance not cure as the primary aim.
This will mean a substantial reordering of priorities in
medical education and medical practice. It also requires
the changing of attitudes of the American people toward
health care. Instead of dependence upon physicians and
other health care providers people should be taught that
the primary responsibility for health lies with themselves,
particularly their habits. Personal life-long behavior
causes many of our current health problems such as excessive
consumption of food and alcohol and cigarette smoking. Early
and more effective education concerning these health risk
factors must be developed, which is the purpose of the
National Health Consumer Information and Health Promotion
Act of 1976. Standards for health education have been developed
by the Bureau of Health Education for educational institutions
such as primary and secondary schools as well as health and
medical care institutions and community health education
programs. Health education needs to concentrate on teaching
individuals to develop an orientation to maintain and protect
optimal function as a fundamental aspect of the preventative
approach to personal health care rather than the current
complaint-response mechanism now utilized by consumers.
Emphasis upon prevention as a national policy should include
education of both the general public and the health professional
in preventive care, and redirection of the payment system
for health services.

The provision of personal health services in the form of

medical care alone is an extremely expensive and not very
productive way of improving community health. The alternatives
of health education, preventative medical services and environmental health programs have not had proportional investments.
Spending for disease prevention and health education represents
3% or less of the total health outlays, with about 2.5% being
spent for prevention and control measures and 0.5% for health
education. Within the federal budget allocations for health
education have increased from ½% in 1973 to 2% in 1977 and
outlays for disease prevention and control are now about 3%
of the health budget. This still falls short of the 10%
which is advocated for disease prevention and health education.[4]
    The American health care system is so complex, however,
and is composed of so many subsystems, and influenced by so
many non-medical institutions that it is unlikely to be substantially altered by a single act of Congress however bold
or venturesome. Even so to solve the current problems calls
for continued study by health professionals and continued
federal support of a variety of programs that address some of
these major concerns. The problems of accessibility for cure of
disease conditions are related to the high cost of such services.
The issue of preventive care and health education likewise will
influence the cost of care.
    A commitment to better health has implications that reach
beyond the medical care system into the very marrow of society
where the origins of health and sickness truly reside. Health
care of the future will call for a judicious mixture of high
technology and home remedies, research and education.
    A comprehensive and accessible health care system is
still a real possibility with almost equal access for all.
To achieve this we must join forces to determine what is the
right amount of health care and who will provide it, at a cost
the nation can afford.

FOOTNOTES

(1) President's Proposal on Hospital Cost Containment
     (H.R. 2626) Hearings Before the Subcommittee on
     Interstate and Foreign Commerce, U.S. House of
     Representatives, Serial 96-19, Part II April 1979.
     U.S. Government Printing Office, Washington, D.C.

(2) Anderson, G., et al. Community Health, C.V. Mosby Company
     1978.

(3) Ibid

(4) Ibid

DISCUSSION SUMMARY: THE RIGHT TO HEALTH CARE

Marc D. Basson

Director, CEHM
University of Michigan
Ann Arbor, Michigan

Participants tended to use the Collins case as a
stimulus to general principles as well as trying to resolve
it on its own merits. The discussion groups' results reflected
this. The discussants were evenly divided on whether a moral
right to health care existed for the general public. Defenders
of such a right argued from the necessity of health for
exercising other moral rights and from general considerations
of social justice. "We are all human beings," explained one
nursing student, " and there should be a societal obligation
to provide for our general welfare." A faculty member from
the School of Public Health added, "It seems to me uncon-
scionable to deny people basic medical care while expending
our resources on personal luxuries."

Opponents were successful in forcing a consensus that
such a right to health care, if it exists, must be limited
and at best prima facie. They argued that such rights may
be analyzed as stemming from an implicit social contract
which demands acceptance of personal responsibilities in
exchange for such rights. They also contended that any
person should have the right to decide for himself whether
to subscribe to such a contractual co-insurance scheme,
especially if it entails supporting other less responsible
or more sickly citizens.

There was a great deal of spirited debate about whether
Collins had a moral right to health care. Supporters noted
that even if there were no general right, Collins's legal
right to health care was created for moral reasons (his
military service) and that Collins was morally entitled

to care because Congress had promised it to him. In response
to objections that Collins's right was contingent upon his
not destroying himself, it was urged that alcoholism is a
disease for which the victim is not responsible.

Opponents of treating Collins contended that while he
might have the disease of alcoholism, he should be forced to
accept treatment for it and to take responsibility for helping
to cure it. Some suggested that Collins be forced into some
treatment program analogous to court-ordered drug addiction
programs. Others felt that it would be inappropriate to
force him to undergo treatment for alcoholism (presumably on
the grounds that he was competent to refuse it) but would
have warned him that he could only be treated in the future
if he were also in an alcoholism program.

**Rights and Responsibilities in Modern Medicine: The Second
Volume in a Series on Ethics, Humanism, and Medicine: 43—45**
© 1981 Alan R. Liss, Inc., 150 Fifth Avenue, New York, NY 10011

INTRODUCTION: LIFE AND DEATH DECISIONS IN THE NEONATAL
INTENSIVE CARE UNIT

Rachel Lipson

Program Director, CEHM
University of Michigan
Ann Arbor, Michigan

While several decades ago he would have probably died,
with today's medical technology the seriously handicapped
newborn has a chance of survival. Unfortunately, he often
has little more, for modern medical treatment does not
guarantee the baby with severe spina bifida or hydrocephalus
a "normal" life, it just offers him the chance to live. The
child has no choice. While some with Down's syndrome or
less serious birth defects may exist happily, other "miracles
of modern medicine" are physically and mentally impaired and
must be cared for by their parents or the state, or both.
Thus, the fate of the defective newborn is now in the hands
of those who may choose whether to keep him alive, and the
question of what should be done for him has many ethical
implications. Does the handicapped child have a right to
life? What sort of life is worth living? What are the
parents' rights and obligations? Who should decide whether
a given child should live? The parents? The medical staff?
An impartial committee? These are just some of the questions
that must be considered in deciding how to act in the neonatal
intensive care unit.

What are the baby's rights? Does he have the right to
live? Professor Smith believes that the child has a right
to life and that this right may be overridden only for the
baby's own benefit. Smith argues that the baby's death is
the best option when it is clear that the child will be
unable to fulfill his need to be happy and his need to be
excellent if he does live. (Smith cautions that happiness
and excellence must be measured in the baby's terms, not
those of the doctors or others caring for him.) Others are

less inclined to give the child the benefit of the doubt.
Michael Tooley (1972), for instance, has argued that the
neonate does not have even a prima facie right to life. He
claims that to have a right to life one must have an idea of
what life is. Accordingly, only beings that possess the
concept of themselves as continuing subjects of experiences
and mental states can have this right. A newborn does not
seem to have these qualities. Thus, both abortion and
infanticide are acceptable in Tooley's terms, and he would
no doubt feel that there was nothing wrong with not treating
a handicapped neonate.

The baby is not the only person whose rights must be
considered in the neonatal ICU. The rights and obligations
of his parents must also be examined, for the parents may
have to bear the burden of caring for a handicapped child
for the rest of their lives. In his paper, Professor Smith
mentions two sorts of arguments. One urges a choice of
death for the baby for the sake of the baby, while the other
does so to protect such other persons as the child's parents.
Smith stresses that these must be distinguished from each
other.

Dr. Fost discusses the issue of parental involvement in
more detail, questioning the reasons for putting the decision
of life or death for the child in the parents' hands. What
gives the mother and father the right to decide? Fost
argues that the parents do not own the child, and that their
rights are not inherently stronger than those of the baby.
Perhaps the parents gain the right to decide because they
are the best proxies for the child. Fost, however, doubts
that this is the case. He explains that the parents have
neither the required medical knowledge nor the ability to
put the baby's best interest before their own, and suggests
that perhaps they should not be involved in the decision-
making process. Others, including Anthony and Iris Shaw
(Shaw & Shaw, 1973), have argued that decisions concerning
the fate of a newborn must be made with some degree of
parental involvement. Thus, the question of who should
decide is still open to debate and must be carefully examined
in making decisions about treating a defective newborn.

Another important issue, one that is involved in all
euthanasia cases, is the distinction between killing and
letting die. Often the arguments for letting die as opposed
to killing seem to lack a strong basis. After all, both

result in the death of the child. John Freeman has argued
(Freeman, 1972) that killing is less painful and more humane.
Yet, Smith urges us to question the character of the person
who would choose to kill rather than allow an infant to die.

Other problems are encountered in arriving at sensible
decisions in the neonatal ICU. Fost attacks the distinction
between ordinary and extraordinary means and argues that it
is meaningless because medical decision-makers often use the
distinction to avoid firm decisions. Fost also stresses the
importance of obtaining the factual material needed to make
an intelligent decision. He points out that the mistakes
that are made are usually the result of unclear information.
The decision to allow a baby's death, however, is not an
easy one, even when as much is known as is medically possible.
Nevertheless, both Fost and Smith shed some light on how such
decisions can be rationally arrived at.

REFERENCES

Freeman JM (1972). Is there a right to die -- quickly?
    J Pediatr 80:904.
Shaw AM, Shaw IA (1973). Dilemmas of "informed consent" in
    children. NEJM 289(17):885.
Tooley M (1972). Abortion and infanticide. Philosophy and
    Public Affairs 2(1):37.

Rights and Responsibilities in Modern Medicine: The Second
Volume in a Series on Ethics, Humanism, and Medicine: 47–48
© 1981 Alan R. Liss, Inc., 150 Fifth Avenue, New York, NY 10011

LIFE AND DEATH DECISIONS IN THE NEONATAL INTENSIVE CARE UNIT

Case for Discussion

Baby Boy Richardson was delivered three-and-a-half months prematurely yesterday, weighing 750 grams. He has not yet been named because it is doubtful whether he will survive The Richardson's pediatrician, Dr. Waring, is not one to mince words. "Your son is in critical condition at the present time. As you know, he was born very early and so his lungs haven't really matured yet. He's breathing, but not well, and even though his lungs may may mature later if he survives they will never be normal. Furthermore, we believe that his brain has probably been seriously damaged by poor oxygenation. Now there's a very remote chance that he could grow up 'normal' but most likely he will be both physically and mentally impaired to some degree, probably severely so. On top of all this, he has developed a pneumonia which could kill him if we don't jump on it with effective antibiotics. I don't want to rub things in, but I want you to know exactly how we stand."

The Richardsons exchange glances silently. They have been trying to have a child for eight years. Sally is 34 years old and she has had two previous miscarriages in this time. Suddenly she asks, "OK, doctor, why are you telling us this again now? What do you want us to do about it?"

"Well," says Dr. Waring hesitantly, "we were wondering what you wanted us to do about it. Or not do, as the case may be."

"What are our choices?" Mr. Richardson asks bluntly.

Dr. Waring pauses and then matches Mr. Richardson's matter-of-fact tone. "If your child were otherwise normal, I would treat his pneumonia with antibiotics. When he spiked a temperature last night, the intern on call did just that, with ampicillin, a good broad spectrum drug. This might control the infection, but I believe there are drugs far more likely to do so. For legal reasons, I would prefer not to stop antibiotic therapy now that it has been started, but I have not yet decided whether to add a more effective drug and would prefer to leave that to you.

"You also have a second choice to make. Your son has esophageal stenosis, which means that nothing can get into his stomach. He is literally starving to death. The surgeons are prepared to operate on this, It is a simple and relatively foolproof operation which I would normally not hesitate to recommend, but in this case perhaps you should think carefully."

Suddenly, Mrs. Richardson interrupts. "You're talking about letting my baby starve to death. Are you crazy? This is my baby, the baby I've been trying to have for years, and I love him no matter what. I want him cared for and cured. I want, oh, I don't know what I want, but I just don't think you can just let a poor innocent baby starve to death."

She bursts into tears and as her husband awkwardly tries to comfort her, he asks, "Isn't there any other less painful way? Couldn't you just give him a shot of something, doctor?"

Doctor Waring frowns. "That sort of thing is strictly illegal, you realize. But, well, I don't particulary care for watching a baby starve to death and I suppose accidents do occasionally happen, if you know what I mean. Personally, I have no more moral objections to killing than to letting die. But my moral objections are not important. This is your son we are discussing. What do you want me to do?"

What are the rights of the child in this situation? What are the rights of the parents? To whom is the doctor obligated and how? What should the Richardsons do?

Rights and Responsibilities in Modern Medicine: The Second
Volume in a Series on Ethics, Humanism, and Medicine: 49—55
© 1981 Alan R. Liss, Inc., 150 Fifth Avenue, New York, NY 10011

DECIDING FOR THE DEATH OF A BABY

David H. Smith

Indiana University

Bloomington, Indiana 47405

I should like to address two distinct but related
topics: first, what are our obligations to very seriously
handicapped or ill children? Second, in what way should we
discharge the radical kinds of obligations we sometimes
have? For the sake of simplicity I shall refer to the first
of these topics as the question of obligation and the second
as the question of character.

I

Let us begin by discussing the question of our
obligations to seriously handicapped newborns. Is it ever
moral to decide not to preserve their lives as long as
possible? I wish to make three remarks about this:

1. When a baby is so seriously handicapped that we think we
should not save him, we should be careful to distinguish two
kinds of arguments or considerations. Some arguments or
considerations urge a choice of death for the sake of the
baby himself: the kind of life open to him would not be
worth living. Other arguments or considerations urge the
same choice so as to protect other persons: siblings,
parents, the health care system or general public -- from
the destructive tensions associated with the handicapped
baby's life. I do not mean to deny the relevance of either
of these kinds of arguments, to pretend that they are or
should be unrelated to each other, or even a priori to claim
that one or another type of argument will always forbid (or
require) a decision for a handicapped infant's death.
Rather, I suggest that the issues must be distinguished for

the sake of clear analysis. There is a great and
understandable tendency to deny that we would let a baby go
for the sake of someone else. That tendency is rooted in
self-deception. Therefore, we should think through both
possibilities in order to see just how far we can take them.
Failure to consider the options at all would be quite
dishonest.

2. Arguments for the baby's death as the best option open
to him raise questions about the fiduciary bonds that bind
us to him. Generally speaking, our fidelity to others means
that we will loyally be concerned with meeting their needs.
Those basic needs fall into two sorts: the need to be happy
and the need to be excellent. Happiness involves freedom
from pain, a sense of security, the possibility of awareness
-- among other things. Of course, no one is ever "perfectly
happy," but happiness is a goal we seek for others. We also
seek excellence for them: we wish them to develop
themselves so as to become good athletes, scholars,
physicians, friends or people.

In this context, I would say that if neither happiness
nor excellence is possible for any person, even a newborn,
then it would be moral to stop trying to save his life. It
is imperative, however, that we not take the kinds of
happiness and excellence that are open to professional
physicians or moralists and measure defective babies against
that standard, for the babies will lose every time. We have
to realize that there are many forms of excellence and
happiness. Thus I find this kind of argument not persuasive
when applied to babies with Down's syndrome and precarious
when applied to babies with anything less than the very most
severe spina bifida lesions. Furthermore, I think we should
remember that newborns, by definition, face an uncertain
future and have no history. It is hard to know how well any
of them will come to terms with life. I think this suggests
giving them the benefit of the doubt. Thus I should say
that very few babies are so "bad" that they should not be
saved. Still, there is such a thing as a life not worth
living, and our loyalty to an infant may require us to let
him out of that, i.e., stop trying to keep him alive.

3. Third, insofar as our consideration of the possibility
of death for the baby is a product of our obligations to
others, that far we must consider questions of justice. Of
course it is fair to ask one person to make sacrifices for

the sake of another; social life requires such exchanges
with some regularity. My presence here deprives my family
in Indiana of my resources; perhaps you would rather say --
Smith's verbosity in Ann Arbor liberates his family! But
the specific issue we face concerns the sacrifice of one
person's (i.e., the baby's) <u>life</u> for the <u>health</u>, wealth, or
happiness of others. Is it <u>fair</u> to ask the baby to make
that degree of sacrifice? Would we ask older persons,
perhaps the senile and aged, to do the same?

Jewish and Christian religious traditions do, often,
allow the killing of one person to protect another, but the
underlying principle in their views has been that the person
whom it is justifiable to kill must be <u>doing</u> something to
another person. He must, in some sense, be <u>threatening</u>
someone. (We can not now get sidetracked into all the
possible meanings of <u>threat</u> in this context.) Because it
was justifiable to kill threateners both capital punishment
and war could, on principle, be defended by these traditions
as forms of protective killing. It is interesting, I think,
to note that it is precisely those forms of killing found
plausible by our intellectual forefathers that are often
least congenial to the modern sensibility. Whereas they
assumed life to be good and could only justify killing as a
<u>public</u> act to <u>protect</u> life, we have so lost confidence in
our forms of political community and the goodness of life
that we find most plausible <u>private</u> acts of killing to bring
an end to <u>suffering</u>.

But I digress. The general point I wish to make about
the protective killing of defective newborns is simply this
-- that handicap and weakness are no reason, in principle,
for a loss of basic human rights. One of those basic rights
a child has is a right to equal respect for his dignity. A
second is equal respect of his right to life. I do not mean
to suggest that he should get all the same forms of care as
others: medical care should be individualized. But we can
not call a society <u>fair</u> if it makes unchecked demands on the
weak. As John Rawls has suggested, it can not be just to
have inequalities that are not to the benefit of the
disadvantaged. If we translate that principle into our
arena it means it can not be fair to withhold treatment from
a baby unless we can say that under the circumstances this
omission is for his benefit. Denial of a right to life
because of defect or weakness is incompatible with social
justice. There are other ways of protecting the parents or

siblings, and care of the retarded is an excellent use of tax and human resources. Thus protective killing of defective newborns is both unnecessary and unjust.

Thus, as we put together our obligations in fidelity to a newborn's needs and our obligations to be fair to him, we see that we can decide to let him go if, and only if, it is in his own interest, i.e., if neither happiness nor excellence is medically possible for him.

II

This apparent euphemism that we should "let some babies go" brings me to the other question I should like to discuss -- it is the question of the character or type of person we are as we do an act. Americans have a great tendency to evaluate everything in terms of consequences or efficiency. There is a none-too-suble utilitarianism about us that pushes us to make all our moral judgments in terms of costs and benefits. In this instinct is revealed a great and tragic limitation of vision.

Let me try to illustrate my point this way. Suppose I were deaf and I had a friend who was a gifted dancer. As we are seated in a room, we see someone coming to the door, and we both want to open it for him. On the radio a ballet score is playing, say, Tchaikovsky's Sleeping Beauty. My friend would dance to the door, pirouetting, leaping, moving all about the room. I would not hear the music and would prosaically walk straight to the door. My course is direct and efficient, while my friend's is indirect and convoluted.

In both cases, there is the same result: a person moves across the room and opens a door; someone enters. One method is more efficient than the other. But it does not follow from these similarities that our actions were identical, or even that the more efficient action was the best one. Quite the contrary, it was my deafness to a whole dimension of reality, my inability to know and to do, that led me to choose the means that I did. My friend and I neither interpret reality in the same way nor do the same things. In both cases, our guest gets in the room, but it seems pretty clear that my friend acted with more style and finesse, in a word, better than I did.

The moral of the story should be clear. In interpreting an action we have to be sensitive to something besides gross, conspicuous consequences. We have to be aware of the significance of form, or style. This matter of form may not be central to the person on whom our act initially falls: in either case, the guest gets into the room. But it is very important with reference to our own integrity and the consequences for patterns of behavior in our culture. A skilled dancer would be untrue to himself if he merely walked unrhythmically to the door -- and he would fail to instruct any novice dancers who happened to be looking on. He must dance because of who he is.

Form or style of action, then, is important for two reasons. First, the form of an act matters to the actor himself. All persons who know the meaning of the word "integrity" are concerned with the mesh, or fit, between their fundamental convictions and their actions. Sometimes this issue is placed in a temporal context. Then we wonder about the consistency of a particular act with past experiences, training or choices. Thus someone might ask about the consistency between a lifelong professional commitment to preserve life and a choice for death, about the compatibility of euthanasia and a medical role or career. Choices can be evaluated in these terms and often with great instructive force.

Nevertheless, I suggest that consistency is not enough. Integrity involves more. We must remember that despicable individuals can be very consistent; so can people at a very low level of moral sensibility. Thus true integrity involves congruity between those fundamental values and commitment we profess and our action. The real gulf the person of integrity spans is not that between the past, or the customary, and the present but between the ideal and the actual. We have integrity insofar as we make our ideals real in our action. Those ideals include a commitment to the life of the weak and helpless.

Second, and consequently, the form of our action is important because through it we teach others. One does not, after all, learn only from the accomplishments of a genius. One is affected, formed and developed by the way people operate. Character is not simply an individual matter, but radiates out, altering in one way or another people who are touched. Therefore the slogan that everybody should do

things in his/her own way is much too simple. If the means
I use to attain my ends are destructive of persons, I should
enact my choice in a different way.

This teaching function of character is rendered all the
more important if we consider one last aspect of my story of
the ballerina. The thing that differentiates me from the
dancer is my tone deafness. I didn't hear the music. Just
so, one can not discern the significance of form, if he
doesn't hear or feel the moral issues involved. Character
can not exist without perception of moral reality. That is
a kind of perception that one learns as one learns
aesthetic judgment -- by example, by listening, by watching
and, to a point, by studying. Once learned, it is a part of
reality. I perceive the world in fundamental moral or
evaluative categories, not just scientific ones. Thus my
assessments or evaluations are fundamentally affected by my
perceptions. My discernment, or lack of it, is of great
moral significance. People without ideals can have no
character.

I go into such detail about this because I think it is
essential if we are to understand the moral difference
between active and passive euthanasia. That distinction
will never make sense to us if we think only in terms of
economic or medical costs and benefits. However, it does
make sense if part of our moral makeup is an ideal that
prohibits killing. Persons sharing such an ideal can not do
acts that are describable as killing, any more than a gifted
dancer can walk as I do. And the ideal remains a valid one.

The implication, of course, is that our perceptions of
of what we do are of great moral significance. Those
perceptions are a product of our culture, of course, but
they are nevertheless part of us. We feel, I think, that
loyalty to the seriously defective requires our care for
them. Passive euthanasia is a letting go, a realization
that life and companionship can only continue at too great
cost to the beloved. Active euthanasia is a hurrying of a
vexatious guest from our territory, a failure of charity.

The difference in these two acts, then, is symbolical.
If you will -- poetic. But it is a difference that matters
-- if not to our patients, to us and to those who learn from
us. We should allow patients to die -- doing all possible,
including heavy analgesic dosages -- to relieve pain. We

should not kill -- with air embolism or KCL. If we fail to
see the difference between these kinds of acts it is as if
we admit we are tone deaf clods in a room full of moral
ballerinas.

III

In summary, I think that we can decide to allow some
newborns to die if we can plausibly say that the choice is
in the best interest of the child -- the best option open to
him. This means adjusting to the kinds of public and family
support that are available; the focus on the specific child
at issue also means that comparisons with other, healthy
children are not to the point. Is no kind of happiness or
excellence possible for this child? If so, and only if so,
a decision for death is a choice of fidelity and justice.
Finally, we should form our choices according to our
discernment or moral sensibility. In rule and example we
should be faithful and teach fidelity to the dying.

Rights and Responsibilities in Modern Medicine: The Second
Volume in a Series on Ethics, Humanism, and Medicine: 57—61
© 1981 Alan R. Liss, Inc., 150 Fifth Avenue, New York, NY 10011

LIFE AND DEATH DECISIONS

Norman Fost, M.D., M.P.H.
Associate Professor of Pediatrics and History
of Medicine, Director, Program in Medical Ethics
University of Wisconsin School of Medicine
Madison, Wisconsin   53792

As a prefatory remark, I hope we don't leave with the
illusion that we are doing a good job with this case. Good
ethics start with good facts, and I don't know the bare
facts that one would need to make a defensible judgement
about this particular child. I don't know his diagnosis;
how old he is; why the doctors think he has brain damage;
and so on. In my experience, 90% of the gross errors we make
in medical-ethical decisions - those which everyone agrees
were wrong in retrospect - went awry because the decision-
makers didn't have their facts straight. That is, information
was readily available which was not sought or considered.
After the decision becomes irreversible, someone says "If we
had only known that, we would have behaved differently".
Our discussion this morning will, therefore, necessarily be
somewhat theoretical. I would like to anchor it to the case,
but we haven't been given the relevant data. There is also
a long list of ethical, legal, and social issues that we
won't get to because of time constraints. I would like to
pick from that list a few things that David Smith didn't
have a chance to address.

There are three commonly used justifications for letting
such infants die, each of which appears inadequate. First
is the distinction between ordinary and extraordinary means.
The argument, in simplest form, states: We have a duty to
use ordinary means to keep a patient alive, but there is no
duty to use extraordinary means. It has widespread intuitive
appeal. It was referred to favorably by the New Jersey
Supreme Court in the Karen Quinlan case.

I would suggest this justification is not only useless but dangerous. The words have no clear meaning which would allow them to be applied to actual cases. If we use undefined words to justify actions, we are simply putting a veneer on decisions that have been made on some other grounds. Some attempt to define ordinary as that which is "natural", implying we have no duty to provide anything that is unnatural. Few neonates would survive if our duty were confined to natural means. Such a definition would relate to the category of "extraordinary means", the heating system in the building, purified water, the pampers, and the prepared milk.

Another definition is based on "undue expense". How much is undue? $1,000? $10,000? $150,000? It is not just the boundary which is vague; I cannot even define a zone of transition. Virtually all hospital care involves expenses which would be a hardship for the majority of families. We wouldn't say an appendectomy, for example, constitutes extraordinary means on the grounds of the expenses being excessive or unbearable for a particular family.

Another way of illustrating the difficulty of defining these terms is to imagine that I were a physician from Mars, beginning practice in your intensive care unit. Suppose my medical skills were sufficient to be on call alone at night, but I asked for guidance on ethical decisions, such as whether to treat a cardiac arrest in a brain-damaged child. If you told me, "Do everything that is ordinary but don't use any extraordinary means", I would ask you to show me the list of which means were ordinary and which were extraordinary. I doubt you would be able to put a single item of technology on either list. If you pointed to the respirator and said that is extraordinary, I would ask "Does that mean the child about to return from the Operating Room, in need of a respirator for a few minutes, need not get it?".

The slipperiness of these terms was exemplified in a survey of pediatricians and pediatric surgeons in the United States and Canada regarding newborns with serious birth defects. Two questions were of special interest: "Would you consider repair of duodenal atresia an ordinary or extraordinary operation?". Nearly all said that would be considered ordinary. They were then asked whether repair of duodenal atresia in a child with Down's Syndrome was ordinary or extraordinary. Most said that would be extraordinary means.

Many doctors who answered the survey were in the odd position of being able to do an operation at 8:00 a.m. on a normal child and say, "I just used ordinary means to keep someone alive", and then at 9:00 a.m., do the identical procedure on a child with Down's Syndrome and say, "I just used extra-ordinary means to keep someone alive". The means couldn't have become extraordinary between 8:00 a.m. and 9:00 a.m. The means were exactly the same. What these respondents apparently meant is that in the case of Down's Syndrome, there was no duty to use even ordinary means to keep the patient alive. That may or may not be true. That is what we are discussing this morning. But if there is justification for withholding treatment from a child with Down's Syndrome, or the child in our case, some other reason has to be found for it other than the means themself. We can't just call the means extraordinary when we don't want to use them and ordi-nary when we do. In the words of Leon Kass, we can't let the technology do the moral work for us.

The second point I want to address is the role of paren-tal involvement in this decision. The majority of pedia-tricians and surgeons involved in these cases believe it is appropriately a matter of parental discretion.[1] There are 3 theories of the parent-child relationship which might underlie this belief. The first would view the parent-child relation-ship as ownership, with the parent possessing the same rights one would have over property. In this view, parental discre-tion is unlimited, and state intervention would be prohibited. It was the prevailing view in western society until the late 19th Century. In England, France, and the United States, parents could abuse their children, and in some places kill them without reprisal. The lack of state response to even gross child abuse persisted until the middle of this century. I think most people no longer believe that the proper relationship between parents and children is described by a notion of ownership. The wide-spread support of child abuse laws are just one indication that we believe the state should intervene when parents are acting in a way that puts their children's lives in jeopardy. An "ownership" doctrine, therefore, can no longer be a justification for letting parents will the death of their children. A second position might be that parents and children are equal in that they both have rights but that the parents have some sort of higher rights or prior rights. It is unclear on what that could be based: Size? Age? Contribution to society? It is espe-cially troublesome when the right that the parents are claiming - to be protected from psychosocial injury which the child may cause them if he lives - is being weighed against the child's right to life. As James Gustafson observed, one person's life cannot be subject to another's desires.[2] We are not here weighing a life against a life, in which case we _might_ prefer the parent's claim.

The third, and probably the most appealing justification for letting parents decide is that they are the best possible proxy for the child. Ideally, if this were a competent adult, we would ask him to decide for himself. But the child can't tell us that so someone has to act in what appears to be the child's best interests. The question is: who is the best person to do that. Many believe the parents are as good as anyone. They are the closest to the child; they have the most invested; they come from the same background; and so on.

There are two minimum conditions for an ideal proxy. First, that they have sufficient knowledge to know what is in the other person's best interest. Second, they should desire and intend to act in the child's best interest, rather than their own. I would suggest most parents lack the necessary knowledge to make an informed judgement in this area. This is not related to intelligence or educational level, but because the shock of having a newborn with a major birth defect or who is critically ill make communication and acquisition of the information very difficult. It is hard enough to teach house officers the facts about these things. To try to get parents to understand the crucial information about the likely benefits and risks of various alternatives is often impossible. I would put involved parents among the lowest groups in the community on this criterion of having the necessary facts to make a decision that would be in the best interest of the child. In that sense, they are poor proxies. I would also question the desire and the intent of some parents to do what is in the child's best interest. When a parent says that they want the child to die because his continued existence would be a threat to them, it appears to me that they disqualify themselves as proxy. This is not because they are evil or bad. I think we should support such parents. But when parents say that they can no longer support the child for emotional or economic reasons, they have abandoned their claim to speak for that child. To put it in a more personal way, if I were in the hospital, seriously ill, are temporarily incompetent and someone had to decide whether I should live or die, the last person I would want to decide is someone who has already said, "If Fost continues to live, it will be a great burden for me".

REFERENCES

1. Shaw A, Randolph JG, Manard B (1977). Ethical issues in pediatric surgery: a national survey of pediatricians and pediatric surgeons. Pediatrics 60:588.

2. Gustafson J (1973). Mongolism, parental desires, and the right to life. Persp in Biol and Med 16:529.

Rights and Responsibilities in Modern Medicine: The Second
Volume in a Series on Ethics, Humanism, and Medicine: 63—64
© 1981 Alan R. Liss, Inc., 150 Fifth Avenue, New York, NY 10011

DISCUSSION SUMMARY: LIFE AND DEATH DECISIONS IN THE
NEONATAL INTENSIVE CARE UNIT

Rachel Lipson

Program Director, CEHM
University of Michigan
Ann Arbor, Michigan

Over ninety percent of the participants in this topic
felt that Baby Boy Richardson had the right to live despite
the fact that he would probably be severely impaired, and
that any treatment which could help keep the baby alive
should be used. Most groups discussed the quality of life
the child could expect and still concluded that he deserved
all possible therapy because, as one participant put it, "if
the child has even a very slight chance of being normal or
slightly abnormal, then he must be operated on. As in many
true neonatal ICU cases," she continued, "there is a chance,
however slight, that Baby Boy Richardson could survive and
grow up normally."

One group based its decision on the belief that society
has an obligation to preserve life. Members felt that while
"the medical knowledge available to the Richardsons is
relevant, it is not sufficient to condemn a child to death."
Those who felt that the child should not be treated argued
that treatment might not be the best thing for the baby.
"Not doing injury is more important than not killing,"
stated one participant. "It may do less harm to this child
to let him die."

Several other issues were also touched upon during the
discussions. Among these was the question of the parents'
rights and obligations. One group felt that the parents had
made their choice in conceiving the child. As one member of
the group said, "In having a child in the first place, the
parents took a chance on its being abnormal, so they are
obligated to care for it and not let it die." Another group

examined Fost's view that the parents are inadequate proxies for the child. They decided, regardless of Dr. Fost's argument, that the parents had to be involved in the decision-making. Some members of the group simply felt that parents know what is best for their own child, while others were concerned about the psychological aftermath and suffering of parents not involved in such a vital decision. A third group emphasized that the parents are also patients of the doctor. Thus, the doctor is obligated to participate in the decision-making process, but, they concluded, must allow them the final say.

Several groups discussed the obligations of the physician in more depth. Most felt that the doctor has a greater obligation to the baby than to the parents. According to members of one group, the doctor must act in such a way as to give the child the best shot at a normal life. Thus, he must operate. One physician argued that if the baby had only a one percent chance at a normal life, then the ninety-nine percent chance of misery probably outweighed this. He claimed that the doctor would be acting in the baby's best interest if he allowed the child to die. The physician was outvoted 10 to 2 in this discussion group's final vote.

INTRODUCTION: ANIMAL RIGHTS AND ANIMAL EXPERIMENTATION

Marc D. Basson

Director, CEHM
University of Michigan
Ann Arbor, Michigan

The seventeenth century philosopher Rene Descartes is
said to have casually thrown a small dog out of his window
to demonstrate his conviction that soulless (i.e., non-human)
animals had the moral status of machines. Certainly our
sentiments about proper treatment of animals have changed
radically since then. Most of us have been taught since
childhood that it is wrong to cause unnecessary pain to
animals. The key to our current beliefs is the word "unnecessary". Most of us would intuitively differentiate
malicious maltreatment from careful scientific experimentation.

Bennett Cohen exemplifies the traditional view that "man
is the measure of all things" and must watch over the rest of
creation. Cohen quotes Dewey approvingly as to man's obligation to use animal experimentation for his own benefit (and
sometimes for the animal's benefit as well). The main theme
of Cohen's paper is man's obligation to "responsible stewardship" of animals and other natural resources. He finds talk
of animal rights "confusing and unconstructive". Yet, it would.
be a serious mistake to dismiss Cohen's position as shallow or
self-justificatory. He is internationally known for his work
in establishing standards for care and treatment of animal
subjects and is deeply troubled by any suggestion that he is
insincere or unconcerned with the welfare of his animal subjects.

Yet, despite Cohen's thoughtfulness and the equal sophis-
tication of his co-speaker, Tom Regan, it is clear that they
never really came to grips with each others' positions. Regan
argues from a totally different ethical framework which accords
rights to anything which feels pain. He appears no more able

to understand and refute Cohen's "speciesism" than Cohen can comprehend animal rights. The reader may be reminded of Thomas Kuhn's comments on the impossibility of rational debate between proponents of competing scientific paradigms.

Regan begins by noting the psychological biases that prejudice us toward our received moral tradition which acknowledges "human rights" and denies those of animals. He argues that a doctrine of moral rights is necessary and that such rights must take precedence over our prejudices and over utilitarian considerations. (This last is plainly an oversimplification which Regan qualifies later, but the simplistic version seems to be implicit in Regan's initial rejection of animal rights for human benefit.)

Regan argues for a "sentience requirement" for moral rights which he interprets to mean that anything that can feel pain has a right not to be hurt. (Note that saying that animals have rights not to be hurt is stronger than saying that it is wrong to hurt animals. Utilitarian considerations, for instance, militate against at least some harm to animals.) Regan cites other possible "requirements" for having rights and argues against them in order to establish his own principle by process of elimination. He does not distinguish between the necessity and sufficiency of feeling pain for having rights.

The reader will have to decide for himself whether he finds Regan's arguments convincing and whether there are alternative principles that Regan does not mention. A social contract theorist, for instance, might tie having rights to the capacity to interact meaningfully with others.

Regan argues separately for the plausibility of granting legal rights to animals. He makes a convincing case for the possibility of doing so, but the reader will have to decide whether it ought to be done. Such legal rights might be justified by the existence of moral rights, or by utilitarian considerations. On the other hand, it may be that, as Bennett Cohen suggests, animals can be adequately protected without creating such legal rights.

Rights and Responsibilities in Modern Medicine: The Second
Volume in a Series on Ethics, Humanism, and Medicine: 67—68
© 1981 Alan R. Liss, Inc., 150 Fifth Avenue, New York, NY 10011

ANIMAL RIGHTS AND ANIMAL EXPERIMENTATION

Case for Discussion

Research on the prevention and treatment of coronary thrombosis (heart attack) has been impeded by the lack of suitable animal models. The condition does not occur often under natural conditions in animals, and the experimental models that have been attempted have not duplicated the human disease very well. This has increased the difficulty of studying the disease and of evaluating drugs that could prevent or limit the severity of heart attacks.

The anti-thrombotic properties of certain drugs have been demonstrated in the test tube. This is the basis for the use of some of these agents in heart attack patients. However, in clinical use, the drugs have not worked as well as the in vitro tests would suggest they should, and some even have had adverse effects. Although the safety of the drugs was tested on animals, their efficacy could not be tested adequately because there has not been a proper model of the human disease. As a consequence, a number of scientists have sought new approaches to the experimental induction and treatment of coronary thrombosis in animals.

Consider the following hypothetical research proposal with respect to the topic of Animal Rights and Animal Experimentation.

Dr. Jones, a pharmacologist and physician, and faculty member at a large research university, proposes to induce coronary thrombosis in 10 rhesus monkeys. His idea is to stimulate a coronary artery continuously for several days with a low level electric current. This stimulation would

damage the coronary artery, cause the blood platelets to concentrate at the point of injury, and would lead to a thrombosis. The stimulation of the artery would not be painful to
the monkeys, but one can infer that at the time the coronary
artery actually thromboses there could be significant pain.
If the validity and reliability of the model could be
established, it would permit evaluation of new drugs for
their ability to prevent or limit the development of thrombosis. The stimulating and recording electrodes would have
to be implanted surgically. The surgical procedure would be
performed using aseptic technique, with the animals under
appropriate anesthesia.

During the post-surgical period and during a second
phase of the project, lasting several months, during which a
series of drugs would be tested, it would be necessary to
permanently maintain the monkeys in restraint chairs. This
is essential to permit continuous recording and monitoring of
heart action during the development of thrombosis. The
response to test drugs also must be evaluated under restraint
since some of them would be given by continuous intravenous
infusion. The restraint prevents the monkeys from damaging
the electrode wires and intravenous catheters. Adequate
veterinary care of the monkeys is assured throughout the
study. They would be observed daily for any physical problems
associated with the restraint and would be given appropriate
veterinary medical treatment as necessary. They would have
adequate access to food and water. However, there would be
no possibility of normal activity. At the conclusion of the
study, the monkeys would be killed with an overdose of
anesthetic to permit microscopic examination of their tissues.

What criteria ought to be used in evaluating the ethical
legitimacy of research such as this? If these animals have
rights, what sorts of rights are they, and to what do
they entitle the monkeys? What circumstances or considerations
would justify violating these rights and to what extent?
Should this research be permitted?

Prepared by Bennett J. Cohen

Rights and Responsibilities in Modern Medicine: The Second
Volume in a Series on Ethics, Humanism, and Medicine: 69–83
© 1981 Alan R. Liss, Inc., 150 Fifth Avenue, New York, NY 10011

ANIMAL RIGHTS AND ANIMAL EXPERIMENTATION

Tom Regan

North Carolina State University

Raleigh, North Carolina

The idea of animal rights is in the air. It is a difficult idea, not only considered philosophically—I shall have
more to say on this score as we proceed—but also psychologically. By this I mean that we have an understandable
resistance to accepting it or even considering it in a
serious light. Our defenses go on alert, as it were, at its
mere mention. And this is true, it seems to me, not only if
our professional life or training happen to put us directly
in contact with animals in ways that bode ill for them, but
also, and more fundamentally, because the idea of animal
rights threatens to crack the window through which, by the
power of custom and culture, we view the world and our place
in it. That view—what, for convenience, I shall call the
received view—is that the world is ours—that it belongs to
us—and that anything else that has value, in addition to
human beings, has it only if (and only so long as) it serves
human purposes, needs, desires or, in a word, human interests.
This view, I believe, is very widespread, and its acceptance
is a source of deep security—(afterall, it tells us that we
not only are valuable; we also are the measure of the value
of all else, in the terrestial sphere at least)—which is
why, as I have said, our defenses come out whenever the received view is challenged, as surely it is by the idea of
animal rights. For the unsettling point behind this idea is
that there are other, non-human individuals who have moral
footing, a moral place in the world, and who have this independently of human interests. Now, if this is true, the
crack appears: We cannot go on viewing the world and our
place in it as the received view decrees. Rationally, we
must change the pane. And it is because most of us, not

just those who use animals in research—it is because most
of us who are products and shapers of Western civilization
accept the received view, I think, that we are challenged by
the idea of animal rights—feel uncomfortable with it and
would like to laugh it out of court, so to speak.

But discomfort with an idea is not sufficient reason to
dismiss it, as history amply demonstrates. No doubt most of
those alive at the time were more secure in viewing the
earth as the center of the physical universe than in re-
ceiving Copernicus' revolutionary idea that the sun is the
center of our solar system. It took courage to think the
unthinkable then. The telescope was not an instrument for
the faint hearted. Or, again—and this time perhaps more
analogously—there is little question that slave owners and
traders felt more secure in viewing human slaves as mere
commodities and were threatened by, felt uncomfortable with,
the thought that slaves had the same rights as owners and
traders did. The fact, then, that we feel at home with one
view, and are uneasy with another, is not by itself sufficient reason to continue to accept the former and to dismiss
the latter. The credentials of each must be examined with a
rational, informed eye, and the final judgment made on the
basis of this examination rather than of habit.

You will understand me when I say that I cannot
possibly conduct a complete examination of the relevant
ideas on the present occasion. Like putting an elephant in
a trunk, the issues just are too large to squeeze into the
space available to me. All that I can hope to do is convey
some sense of the landscape regarding the debate over animal
rights. I shall do this by first giving a rough comparison
of moral and legal rights. Then I shall examine arguments
for and against ascribing these rights to animals. In conclusion I shall return to the point from which I have begun
—the impact of animal rights on what I have called the received view.

I. Moral Rights and Legal Rights

A right can be understood as a valid claim the pos-
sessor has against another. To illustrate: If I have a
right to an inheritance, then I cannot only claim that the
inheritance is mine—(I am not only empowered to say that it
is mine)—I am justified in taking certain steps to see that

I actually get it—(my claim, that is, is valid). By contrast, persons who do not have a right to an inheritance may
claim it is theirs but, lacking any right to it, they are
not justified in taking steps to get it. Their claim is not
valid.

What gives validity to anyone's claim? This can and
does vary. In particular this varies depending on whether
one is speaking of moral rights or legal rights, since legal
rights acquire their validity from the law, while moral
rights, if there are such, acquire their validity from the
principles of an enlightened morality. Both ideas need to
be explained more fully, beginning with the idea of legal
rights.

It is clear that the laws of one country frequently
differ from the laws of another. In the United States, for
example, it is unlawful (normally) to drive on the left; not
so in England. The explanation of this variability is
simple: Laws are created by the legislative acts or decrees
of various persons living in various countries at various
times, and, like other creative activities, the products of
this one—namely, laws—are bound to differ. Similarly in
the case of the legal rights of the citizens of these
countries: What legal rights citizens have also is a matter
of legislation or other legally authorized decrees; and these,
too, can and do vary from nation to nation. Moreover, because legal rights are made by humans, they can also be un-
made. What was once a matter of legal right in a particular
country can cease to be so, as, for example, slave owners in
the United States once had the legal right, based on property
rights, to buy and sell slaves.

The idea of a moral right differs in important respects
from that of a legal right. First, moral rights are supposed to be universal; that is, if any individual (A) has a
moral right (for example, a moral right to life), then all
other individuals like A in the relevant respects also have
this right, no matter where these other individuals live, or
when, and no matter what the laws of their country happen to
be. Second, moral rights, unlike legal rights, are not the
result of human creative activity; they are not "brought into existence" by democratic vote, the whim of a despot, etc.
Rather, moral rights are discovered, not in the way, say,
continents or black holes are discovered—not by doing
empirical science, for example—but by thinking hard about

moral questions. Like basic postulates in science, moral rights, if there are any, are what reason compels us to postulate, if we are to give the most satisfactory theoretical account of morality. Needless to say, this "discovery" of moral rights is a long story, one that cannot be recounted here, though later on, when the position known as utilitarianism is discussed, a rough sketch of some parts of the story will be offered. Suffice it to say that, if there are moral rights, they are unlike legal rights: The latter are created by humans; the former are not.

A final defining characteristic of moral rights is that they are equal. This means that if any two individuals, A & B, both have the same moral right, then both possess this right equally. No one person's moral right can be greater than any other's. Thus, for example, whites do not have greater moral rights than blacks, men than women, adults than children, Americans than Viet Cong, etc. When it comes to moral rights, all who have them are equal.

Now, the rights enshrined in the Declaration of Independence—the rights to life, liberty, and the pursuit of happiness—frequently are cited as examples of moral rights. This is intelligible. For suppose that a particular government instituted and enforced laws that discriminated against certain citizens on the basis of skin color, sex, or religious affiliation. Suppose those discriminated against were arbitrarily killed or denied the freedom to emigrate. Than, if we wanted to object to this discrimination, we could not argue that it was unlawful since, in that country, it is not. Legally, everything is above board. Rather, we would have to couch our objection in moral terms, and one way we might voice it is by charging that the government was violating the moral rights of some of its citizens.

Not everyone is agreed that there are moral rights. The arguments for and against them are complex and varied. However, one attempt to dispense with moral rights needs to be characterized, both because it is a widely held and influential view and because its apparent shortcomings help to highlight the importance of moral rights. The attempt in question is the position known as utilitarianism. In fact, this single word, 'utilitarianism', is not the name of a single position; there are many different positions that can be and are referred to as utilitarian. What they all have in common is their emphasis on the consequences (the results

or effects) of actions or rules of action, including legislation. What they all say is that the morality of an action
or rule depends entirely upon how valuable the consequences
are, a morally right act being one which, roughly speaking,
brings about more good than would have resulted had any
other act been performed, while a morally wrong act is one
that brings about more evil (e.g., more pain or suffering)
than would have resulted if another alternative had been
chosen. Moral rights, in the sense under discussion, are,
according to this theory, superfluous; there is no good
reason to postulate them and very good reason not to.

Now, the major difficulty all forms of utilitarianism
encounter is that they all seem to be committed to the view
that the end justifies the means. So long as the results of
a certain action or rule bring about the best consequences,
the action or rule are above moral criticism, according to
the utilitarian. But the problem with this way of thinking
is that acts or rules that are flagrantly wrong might emerge
as morally quite all right. A standard example is that of
slavery. Might it not be the case that an economy based on
slavery brought about the best consequences, all considered,
in, say, nineteenth century America? If so, then utilitarians seem necessarily to be committed to supporting slavery
under those conditions. Critics of utilitarianism, on the
other hand, think we ought to condemn slavery, even if it
happens to be the best economic system. But if we do not
accept the utilitarian's position, how might we attempt to
explain why slavery is wrong? Enter the idea of moral rights:
It is because human beings each have certain moral rights
(e.g., to life and liberty), and because these rights are
universal and equal, that, according to these thinkers, it
cannot be morally justifiable to treat some human beings,
against their will, in ways that it would be wrong to treat
others. Thus, if we think it would violate the rights of
whites to enslave them in order to bring about the best consequences, then, given that whites and Blacks have equal
moral rights, enslaving Blacks for similar reasons also
would violate their rights. Those who argue for moral
rights, therefore, think that positions such as utilitarianism, which attempt to dispense with these rights, are inadequate. And although many of the details and subtleties
of this debate have gone undiscussed on the present occasion,
hopefully enough has been said to suggest why the idea of
humans having moral rights is an important one.

Utilitarianism will be briefly considered again later on. For the present, suppose we were to grant that human beings do have certain moral rights, in particular the three rights enshrined in the Declaration of Independence. These, then, are rights possessed equally by human beings, whatever their race, religion or sex, and independently of what their nation's laws happen to say. Two further questions can then be explored. First, we can inquire into the <u>grounds</u> of these rights: We can ask what there is about human beings that can serve as the basis of their possessing moral rights. And, second, we can go on to examine how alternative answers to this first question impinge on the debate over whether animals have moral rights. These are the issues to which I shall now turn my attention.

II. Do Animals Have Moral Rights?

What are the grounds of human possession of moral rights? Various answers have been proposed. A cursory examination of some of the most important follows.

> The <u>Species</u> <u>Requirement</u>: This view
> states that all and only members of
> the species homo sapiens have moral
> rights. Thus, since all humans and
> no animals are members of this species,
> all humans have moral rights but all
> animals lack them.

This requirement can be challenged in a variety of ways, but one stands out. The Species Requirement implies that moral questions can be answered by biological considerations—in this case, species membership. However, prejudices such as racism and sexism also attempt to answer moral questions on biological grounds, in their case by appeals to race or sex. If, as is agreed, these latter positions are morally unacceptable, the suspicion arises that the same is true of the view espoused by the Species Requirement: It, too, expresses a morally unacceptable prejudice (what many now call "speciesism")—namely, a prejudice against members of species other than our own. To make this clearer, imagine this possibility: Beings from another planet (extraterrestrials) pay earth a visit. They are intelligent, display the ability to remember and imagine, feel pleasure and pain, are able to communicate, have preferences and, in a word, are like "normal" humans when it comes to their abilities. However, despite these noteworthy similarities, they do not have moral rights, according to the Species Requirement. Why? Not because humans are able to do some things these extra-terrestrials can't. Rather, it is because humans happen to belong to the "right" species. But this surely is rank pre-judice, comparable in terms of its pernicious logic to rac-ism and sexism, where various individuals are denied rights because they do not belong to the "right" race or sex. The Species Requirement, therefore, is inadequate.

> The Rationality Requirement: This
> view holds that all and only ration-
> al beings have moral rights. Thus,
> even extraterrestrials have moral
> rights, if, as supposed in the pre-
> ceding, they are rational. Animals,
> however, since they are not rational,
> do not have moral rights.

Two objections to this view will suffice. First, it is not clear that animals cannot reason. On the contrary, many, many animals appear to be able to do so. Accordingly, if we were to accept the Rationality Requirement, many animals would have moral rights. But, second, like the Species Re-quirement, the Rationality Requirement is not adequate. For there are many human beings who are not rational; for ex-ample, severely mentally enfeebled humans and the mentally deranged are not. However, if all humans have moral rights, these humans have moral rights. And if they have moral rights and yet are not able to reason, then the ability to reason cannot be a requirement individuals must meet in order to have moral rights.

> The Modified Species Requirement: This
> requirement states that all and only
> those individuals who belong to a
> species whose members typically (or
> normally) are rational have moral rights.
> Thus this requirement does not include
> only sapiens; even extraterrestrials can
> have moral rights, if the typical mem-
> bers of their species are rational. The
> Modified Species Requirement thus is not
> open to the principal objection raised
> against the Species Requirement. More-

> over, mentally enfeebled and deranged
> humans also have moral rights, given
> the Modified Requirement, since they
> belong to a species (homo sapiens)
> whose members are normally or typically
> rational. Thus, this requirement also
> overcomes the principal objection rais-
> ed against the Rationality Requirement.
> Animals, however, come out on the short
> end again, since they do not belong to
> species whose members normally or typ-
> ically are rational.

The apparent success of this requirement is just that:
Apparent. For, first, if it is true that some animal species
do normally or typically have members that are rational,
then all members of these species will have moral rights,
given the Modified Species Requirement. Thus, for example,
all members of species of primates would seem to qualify as
possessors of moral rights. But, second, the case of our
extraterrestrials needs to be reconsidered. The ones who
visit the earth are rational, we have supposed; only now
imagine that they are the abnormal ones, so far as their
species is concerned; that is, the members of their species
normally or typically are not rational. This being so, we
would be compelled to deny that our visitors had moral rights,
given the Requirement under examination, not because of any
fault of their own, not because they were unable to do something normal humans were able to dc, but merely because of
some fact about the species to which they happen to belong.
This is palpably unfair. Whatever else may be unclear or
uncertain about moral rights, it at least is clear and certain that no one individual can lack moral rights because of
what is true of some other individual(s).

A general theme emerges from the inadequacy of the preceding requirements. It is that moral rights, because they
are possessed by individuals, must be based on what is true
of the individuals who possess them and that the requirement
for possessing moral rights must not exclude those humans who
are enfeebled, or deranged. This is why many have thought
that the next requirement is the most adequate. It is

> The Sentience Requirement: All and only
> individuals who are sentient (that is,
> can experience pleasure and pain) have

          moral rights. Thus, deranged and
          enfeebled humans have moral rights.

     Now, not everything is smooth sailing even for this re-
quirement. In particular the moral status of irreversibly
comatose human beings poses a quite serious problem, since,
given the Sentience Requirement, these humans have no moral
rights. However, this does not mean that we would be morally entitled to do anything we like to these humans. On the
contrary, it is open to anyone who accepts the Sentience Requirement to insist that we are always to treat all humans
with respect, even those who are irreversibly comatose, because (a) we may not know that they are in an irreversible
state and thus may not know that they lack moral rights, and
because (b) we ought always to act in ways that promote respect for human life, and showing respect for comatose humans,
even those who are irreversibly so, is one way to foster this
respect. In these ways, then, those who accept the Sentience
Requirement might defend their position against objections
based on considerations about irreversibly comatose human
beings. And to the extent that these defenses are adequate,
to that extent at least a very strong case can be made for
the adequacy of this requirement.

     Now, if the Sentience Requirement passes the tests of
its adequacy, a rational basis is provided for enfranchising
many, many animals in the class of individuals possessing
moral rights. For there are many, many animals who are
sentient. Granted, where we draw the line between those who
can feel pain and those who cannot is uncertain. But there
can be no reasonable doubt that many animals can feel pain
or that many of the animals routinely used by humans as a
source of food and in research, in science fairs and in
classroom demonstrations, because they are sentient, would
qualify as possessors of moral rights.

     From the moral point of view, therefore, we must seri-
ously inquire into the justifiability of using animals in
these ways. And one central truth about moral rights must
be kept in mind, if our earlier remarks about utilitarianism
are correct: This is that we cannot justify overriding the
moral rights of some just so we can bring about good results
for others. In other words, we cannot justify overriding
moral rights because others will receive some positive good,
either in a human case, such as that of slavery, or in the
case of our use of animals.

Perhaps someone will suggest that the case of animals is different, that our use of them <u>can</u> be justified because it benefits us, whereas our use of other humans <u>cannot</u>. And doubtless many people believe this. The challenge these people must meet is to give good reasons for thinking this true, a challenge compounded all the more by the fact that the animals in question resemble enfeebled human beings in at least one crucial respect—namely, both are sentient. Thus, if we think it would violate the rights of these humans to use them in, say, research, it is unclear at best to see how we are not violating the moral rights of these animals by using them in these ways. The importance of the idea of the moral rights of animals in part is due to its role in forcing us to come to terms with the morality of the ways we routinely treat animals. It is also important because it is relevant to the related issue of granting legal rights to animals, an issue to which we shall now turn.

III. Should Animals Have Legal Rights?

Though many people apparently think otherwise, animals do not now have legal rights. True, they are protected by various laws, such as anti-cruelty legislation and the Endangered Species Act. But buildings and works of art also are protected by laws; yet they do not have legal rights. Indeed, so far as the law is currently written and understood, animals are in the same general legal category as buildings and works of art. Like them, animals are not "legal persons." And since only legal persons can possess legal rights, animals do not possess legal rights.

Even granting that animals are not <u>now</u> accorded the status of legal persons, it does not follow that they cannot or should not be given this status in the future. To begin with, "persons" within the law are not restricted to human beings. Ships and corporations, for example, are legal persons. Thus, in arguing that animals ought to be accorded the status of legal persons, one is not asking the law to perform a biological trick: One is not asking the law to change animals into human beings! Moreover, if we ask what characterizes legal persons, a strong case can be made for placing animals in this category and removing them from the legal limbo they presently share with buildings and works of art.

The following ideas characteristically are attributable to legal persons:

- Legal persons can be injured.
- Legal persons can be benefitted.
- Legal persons have interests.

Now, whereas there is no literal sense in which, say, a building can be injured, benefitted, or have its interests represented, respected or ignored, the same is not true in the case of those animals who are sentient. For these animals do have an interest in avoiding pain; they can be injured; and they can be benefitted. There is, then, no logical bar to granting the status of legal person to these animals.

In reply it might be argued that since legal rights are valid claims, and since animals cannot claim anything, therefore they cannot have legal rights. This objection fails to hold. Ships cannot claim anything; corporations cannot claim anything; yet these "individuals" have legal rights. Animals, therefore, cannot be denied legal personhood because of their inability to make claims. Furthermore, enfeebled humans often are unable to make claims, and yet the law also recognizes that others, acting on behalf of the interests of the enfeebled, can claim what is due them as a matter of legal right. This being so, there is no compelling reason for denying that others, acting on behalf of the interests of animals, could make and press those claims which the animals themselves are incapable of making, pressing or, again like the enfeebled, even understanding.

Still, even if animals could be accorded the status of legal persons, could be accorded legal rights, the question remains, Ought we to do so? Now, this question would be of theoretical interest only, if we had good reason to believe that present and forthcoming legislation already respects and protects the interests of animals. If it did, then making animals legal persons, and giving them legal rights, would be superfluous. But the law is not so good at respecting and protecting the interests of animals as to make the call for granting them rights superfluous, as witness, for example, this not untypical ruling of the New Mexico Supreme Court on the legality of cock-fighting.

While it is true that in the minds of

some men, there is nothing more
violent, wanton, and cruel, necessarily producing pain and suffering to an animal, than placing
a cock in a ring with another cock,
both equipped with artificial spurs,
to fight to the death, solely for
man's amusement and sport, others
consider it an honorable sport mellowed in the crucible of time so as to
become an established tradition not
unlike calf-roping, steer riding, bull-
dogging, and bronco busting.

What this ruling illustrates so well is that the law allows human interest to be the measure of the legality of
practices involving animals, independently of how these
practices affect the interests of the animals themselves.
The court in this case weighs the interests some humans have
in avoiding cruelty, etc., against the interests other humans
have in preserving one among a number of sports "mellowed in
the crucible of time." Nowhere is there any mention of
whether cock-fighting is in the interests of the chickens—or
bull dogging in the interests of the bulls, etc. Nor will
there be such consideration, so long as animals are denied
the status of legal persons.

How, then, might we argue on behalf of animals in this
regard? The following argument merits consideration.

1. The law already allows that non-
humans can be legal persons; therefore, there is no reason why animals
cannot have this legal status.
2. The law already accords legal rights
to mentally enfeebled humans.
3. Sentient animals are similar to enfeebled humans both in terms of
their sentience and because the
case for postulating moral rights in
the case of these humans is just as
strong as the case for postulating
them in the case of these animals
(see Part II, above).
4. The law ought to treat similar cases
similarly.

5. Therefore, the law ought to treat
    animals similarly to the way it
    treats enfeebled humans.
6. Therefore, the law ought to accord
    legal rights to sentient animals.

Whether this argument can withstand the test of informed
criticism cannot of course be decided on this occasion. But
it does serve to illustrate how one might argue for granting
legal rights to animals independently of appeals to sentiment
or to how "cuddly" animals are, since, presumably, no one will
suggest that roosters or bulls make cuddly companions. The
issue is one of fact and reason, not of "mere sentiment."

The legal status of animals used in research would have
to change, if this argument, or another better one, could be
made on behalf of granting legal rights to them. Present
state and federal laws relating to research animals, including the Federal Laboratory Animal Welfare Act (1966), the
Animal Welfare Act (1970) and its amendments (1976), cover
only the transportation, procurement and care of animals;
they expressly exempt the treatment animals receive in research itself. Indeed, this legislation expressly leaves to
the researchers the decision as to when research has begun
and when it has ended. In the words of the 1966 Act, "(t)he
important determination of when an animal is in actual research (and so is not covered by this legislation)...is left
to the research facility." Thus, while subsequent legislation strengthened the 1966 Act and increased the number of
species and animal-related activities covered by this legislation, actual scientific research remained a legislative
taboo. It was and is a matter of self policing, with no
legal sanctions for abuse and no legal procedures for report-
ing it.

This will have to change, if the case for the legal
rights of animals can be made. Legally, (and morally for
that matter), it is a grievious error to authorize the very
persons who can abuse animals used in research to judge
whether abuse occurs, just as legally, (and morally for that
matter), it would be a grievious error to authorize parents
themselves to determine when and if child abuse occurs.
Precisely what form of protection animals used in research
should enjoy, and what procedures should ensure their protection, these are matters that are unclear to me. They pose
very difficult questions. The more modest point I want to

insist upon is that they pose legitimate ones.

Two points in closing. The first reiterates a point
made at the outset—the idea that talk of animal rights
assaults the view that the world is ours and that what has
value, in addition to human beings, is what serves our interests. Earlier I said that the idea of animal rights challenges this view because, if accepted, it would commit us to
regarding animals as having value independently of whether
they serve these interests. Why is this? Very roughly, I
think it is because, when we go deeper into the idea of
animal rights, it is not merely the fact of sentience that
is crucial; it is because what we do to animals matters to
them individually—because it contributes to or detracts
from the quality of their life—that they are meaningful
possessors of rights. It is, I think, not only because they
are alive, but because they have a life that is more or less
valuable to them, individually, logically independently of
whether they serve our interests, that makes attributing
rights to them intellectually intelligible and morally imperative. That we are not accustomed to viewing animals in
this light; that, in fact, we have great difficulty in thinking of them as having value except as they meet our needs or
further our purposes; that, I think, is both regrettable and
correctible. The "correctible" part will take a long time
nonetheless.

Second, and finally, it would be easy to misunderstand
my position. It would be easy to read it as (to use an out-
dated, emotion-packed terminology) "absolute anti-vivisec-
tionism." This would be to misinterpret what I have argued.
For though I have argued for animal rights, both moral and
legal, given certain assumptions, it does not follow that I
must think that any use made of any animal in any experiment
is wrong—a violation of the animal's right—anymore than,
if I had argued for our right to free speech, I would be
committed to thinking that it is quite all right to shout
"Fire!" in a crowded theater. Rights, in other words, though
a very weighty, are not always the only, morally relevant
consideration. There are, I think, circumstances that can
and do arise that would justify us in overriding an individual's right. What these circumstances are—or, more importantly, what the principles are that specify what these circumstances are—these matters are too large for a short survey like the present one. All that can be hoped is that the
preceding has made a case for thinking that those who would

use animals in research are the ones who must justify doing so, if and as the rights of animals are involved.

**Rights and Responsibilities in Modern Medicine: The Second
Volume in a Series on Ethics, Humanism, and Medicine: 85—92**
© 1981 Alan R. Liss, Inc., 150 Fifth Avenue, New York, NY 10011

ANIMAL RIGHTS AND ANIMAL EXPERIMENTATION[1]

Bennett J. Cohen

Unit for Laboratory Animal Medicine

University of Michigan, Ann Arbor, MI 48109

INTRODUCTION

The participants in this Conference are a unique multi-
disciplinary group. The organizers have encouraged attend-
ance by philosophers, lawyers, legislators, religious author-
ities, teachers, biological scientists, veterinarians, physicians, ancillary health care personnel, and a sizable
number of University students. Given our varying back-
grounds of education, experience, and interests, it is certain that our discussion will be wide-ranging, and will reflect many points of view. There is, however, unity in our
diversity, in our respective commitment to the truth and to
the search for rational approaches to the ethical problems
we have been asked to address. This conception of unity in
diversity has guided my preparations for this program.

Professor Regan and I share the task of introducing the
discussion. We are to state our respective approaches to
the question of animal rights and animal experimentation,
and to provide background information to aid consideration
of the case before us. My position can be stated briefly as
follows: I support animal experimentation for three fundamental reasons: it is scientifically valid and ethical; it
is essential to the development of new knowledge in biology
and medicine; and, it contributes to the welfare of human
beings and other animals. In this context, man's relations
with other animals involve responsible stewardship, not

[1]Presented at the Fourth Conference on Ethics, Humanism,
and Medicine, November 10, 1979, Ann Arbor, Michigan

"animal rights", a term that I find both confusing and unconstructive in relation to the use of animals in research.

Before commenting specifically on the case before us,
I wish to pose and attempt to answer three questions which
I believe will place the ethical issues in an appropriate
context for our subsequent discussion: 1) are there alternatives to animal experimentation; 2) is humane use of animals in research a contradiction in terms; and 3) what protection do animals have against abuse in laboratories?

ARE THERE ALTERNATIVES TO ANIMAL RESEARCH?

The concept of alternatives to animal research has become popular among critics and opponents of animal experimentation in recent years. Animal welfare organizations
are espousing the cause with increasing dedication. In
England, an organization called FRAME (Fund for the Replacement of Animals in Medical Experiments) has been promoting
the concept for more than ten years. In this country,
HR 4805 has been introduced in the 96th Congress to create
a National Center for Alternative Research. If the bill
becomes law, from 30-50% of all federal appropriations for
animal research would have to be directed to the development of alternative methods. Well-organized efforts are
underway to convince the public and legislators that studies
involving live animals no longer are needed or could be
greatly limited, that mathematical models, computer programs,
tissue culture methods, and chemical tests are effective
alternatives to the use of animals in research.

The idea that scientists are unaware of or, somehow,
are reluctant to use readily available alternatives to animals is false--a nonissue if ever one existed. In the real
world of medical and biological science, a decision to use
or not to use animals is made on very pragmatic scientific
grounds. Hypothesis development and testing is the name of
the game. This is how progress is made. It requires employment of the best available methods, whatever those methods may be. Sometimes the use of animals may be an absolute
requirement, as for example in evaluating drug efficacy and
safety or in studying certain aspects of the pathology of
aging. Sometimes other approaches that do not require use
of animals may be appropriate, as for example, the use of
cell culture systems to study the contribution of microsomes

to cell function. The issue is not "alternatives", but how best to search for answers to properly posed scientific questions. It is unfortunate that some critics of animal research are blind to this fact of scientific life and are hateful and unreasoning in their commentary on the so-called "alternatives" issue. I shall not say more about the extremist fringe because, as Dr. Sam Shuster stated in his review of the book Alternatives to Animal Experiments (Shuster, 1978), "Absolute refutation of absolute nonsense is absolutely impossible." It is more important to deal with the legitimate ethical concerns of moderates among animal welfarists, including many medical and biological scientists, who recognize the need for animal research, but who want to be sure that humane considerations are part of the equation.

More than 50 years ago, John Dewey put the case for animal experimentation as follows: "Scientific men are under definite obligation to experiment upon animals so far as that is the alternative to random and possibly harmful experimentation upon human beings, and so far as such experimentation is a means of saving human life and of increasing human vigor and efficiency. The community at large is under definite obligations to see to it that physicians and scientific men are not needlessly hampered in carrying on the inquiries necessary for an adequate performance of their important social office of sustaining human life and vigor." (Dewey, 1926). Except that Professor Dewey did not acknowledge that other animals as well as human beings benefit from animal research, and that women as well as men participate in science and should not be hampered needlessly, his statement is as relevant today as it was in the early 1920s. More recently, Dr. Maurice Visscher has argued that "the use of both human and animal subjects under proper conditions is not only ethically justified, but there is a moral imperative to carry out such studies in an ethical society." (Visscher, 1975). Professor Dewey and Dr. Visscher have recognized as I believe all of us should, that the scientific method, of which animal research is an important component, is an essential instrument of enlightenment and societal progress. In this sense, there are no alternatives to animal research.

IS HUMANE USE OF ANIMALS A CONTRADICTION IN TERMS?

Peter Singer, the philosopher of animal liberation, has

argued strongly that most, if not all, animal research involves the infliction of suffering on non-humans for trivial
purposes. He classifies most humans as "speciesists"--peo-
ple who allow the interests of their own kind to override
the greater interests of members of other species. He op-
poses the so-called "tyranny of human over non-human animals" (Singer, 1975). In other words, the humane use of
animals in research is a contradiction in terms.

I disagree with Singer. Far from being trivial, most
animal research has highly significant purposes. It is
carefully reviewed for scientific merit before being under-
taken. It serves the important societal purpose of developing new knowledge with the ultimate objective of alleviating
pain and suffering. To argue that animal research adds to
the world's pain and is inherently inhumane or immoral, is a
gross distortion of the truth. One may ask, as Maurice
Visscher has, whether views such as this are not in themselves immoral, since they would impose unnecessary and un-
desirable impediments to research (Visscher, 1975). That
some animals experience pain or discomfort during experimentation, or that some experiments may prove to be trivial,
cannot be denied. The remedy for these problems, however,
does not lie in restricting animal studies, as Singer would
advocate. The remedy lies in generating increased understanding and agreement among scientists about the elements
of humane animal care and use, accompanied by specific programs to implement those elements.

The elements of human treatment of animals are not
philosophical concepts; but very specific processes and procedures. They include proper design of experiments; adequate housing and husbandry methods; continuing evaluation
of the animals' health status; provisions for adequate veterinary care, including the appropriate use of anesthetics,
analgesics, and tranquilizers; supportive measures to mini-
mize pain or discomfort in surgical and non-surgical aspects
of research; and the use of appropriate methods of killing
animals when a study is completed. The skills and training
of the personnel in these aspects of humane treatment also
are significant. When these elements are dealt with adequately, the humane use of animals turns out to be a practical, attainable objective. The scientific community is
strongly committed to humane treatment of animals not only
because it is an ethical imperative, but also because it is
an important control factor in research. Certainly, it is
not a contradiction in terms.

WHAT PROTECTION DO ANIMALS HAVE AGAINST ABUSE IN LABORATORIES?

I alluded earlier to the concept of responsible stewardship of animals in research and to the consequent responsibility for the practical implementation of humane treatment procedures. Responsible stewardship also implies acceptance by the scientific community of certain ethical principles such as the research should offer the possibility of fruitful results for the good of society; it should be based on adequate knowledge of the disease or problem under study; it should be conducted so as to avoid unnecessary suffering or injury; it should include provisions for treatment of the animals in accordance with acceptable practices in veterinary medicine; and it should include provisions for terminating an experiment whenever its continuation could lead to unnecessary injury or suffering.

During the past generation, a broad range of standards, policies, and laws have evolved to guide and regulate animal experimentation. All of them protect animals against abuse. There are, of course, general laws against cruelty to animals in all 50 states. These laws are applicable against wanton cruelty in a laboratory setting as well as on a public street or in a private home. I have worked in major research universities all of my professional life, since graduating from veterinary school nearly 30 years ago. I have never witnessed or heard of wanton abuse of an animal in a research laboratory that would qualify for prosecution under the general law against animal cruelty. There are significant problems and deficiencies in the use and care of animals in some laboratories; but wanton cruelty is not one of them. The major problems and deficiencies stem from unawareness, lack of training, poor facilities, inadequate experimental design, and so forth. The remedies are available in the regulatory process that now exists, and, more importantly, in the programs now extant in most scientific institutions to assure adequate care of laboratory animals.

The Animal Welfare Act has set minimum standards for procurement, housing, transportation, and veterinary care of dogs, cats, rabbits, guinea pigs, hamsters, non-human primates, and certain other species. Institutional compliance is evaluated by federal inspectors during unannounced visits on a regular basis. Michigan and other states have enacted similar laws which supplement and complement the federal law.

The scientific community itself has made a powerful
contribution to upgrading standards and practices in the use
and care of animals. Since 1965, the American Association
for Accreditation of Laboratory Animal Care (AAALAC) has
been accrediting scientific institutions that meet the standards of the Guide for the Care and Use of Laboratory Animals
(1978). The Guide is a compendium of recommendations on good
practice in the care and use of animals. The recommendations
are based on experience and scientific principles and they
constitute a definition of humane treatment of animals in
professional terms. Hundreds of institutions now participate
in the AAALAC program, and hundreds of thousands of copies
of the Guide have been distributed since its initial publication in 1963. The National Institutes of Health has played
an important role in generating support for AAALAC and the
Guide. It has issued its own guidelines requiring grantee
institutions to provide written assurance of their compliance
with the standards in the Guide (1979). Maintenance of
AAALAC accreditation is one of the acceptable methods of
assuring compliance. Failure to provide the necessary assurance statement could result in the loss of grant funds, and
this is a powerful incentive in generating institutional
cooperation.

In most scientific institutions, animal care programs
now operate under veterinary direction. Indeed, the adequacy of animal care must be certified by a veterinarian in
all institutions that are required to register under the
Animal Welfare Act. Most institutions also have a standing
committee on use and care of animals which establishes appropriate guidelines and provides an institutional mechanism for monitoring use. Finally, virtually all scientific
journals have policies that bar the publication of research
that is deemed inhumane by the reviewers. It is evident,
therefore, that an effective structure of laws and standards
exists to prevent abuse of animals and to foster better care
of animals in research laboratories.

PRELIMINARY COMMENTS ON THE CASE FOR DISCUSSION

I turn attention now, briefly, to the case for discussion. It deals with research on coronary thrombosis, a
major medical and social problem, for which completely adequate control, treatment, or preventive measures are not yet
available. The extent of the problem can be highlighted by

the following numbers. In the United States it is the leading cause of death among 20-64 year old men; the median age
of males dying suddenly is 59. The death rate is about one
per minute, or more than 1200 per day. In about 25% of the
cases there are no prior symptoms before the fatal attack.
It is readily understandable why this disease problem should
be a focus of scientific interest and study.

As we now consider the criteria for determining the
permissibility or nonpermissibility of the proposed research
involving rhesus monkeys, a series of questions come to mind
that I assume Dr. Jones himself would have considered in
planning his project. Certainly, questions like the ones I
shall list in a moment would be raised during merit review
of the project before funding. I know that I would want to
examine the answers before deciding whether the research
should or should not be permitted. Given only the description of a project which clearly involves exposure of a species
closely related to man to significant pain and distress, I
would have to reserve judgment on permissibility pending
satisfactory answers to the following questions:

1. What is the scientific justification for selecting
   rhesus monkeys for this research?
2. Has similar research been done using other species?
   What is the bearing of any such research on this project?
3. What is the evidence that the proposed procedure of
   electrical stimulation of the coronary artery to produce
   thrombosis would be successful?
4. What would be the fate of the monkeys if the thrombosis
   procedure does not work as projected?
5. Why is there no mention of the use of analgesics in con-
   junction with the development of thrombosis?
6. Have Dr. Jones and his staff worked previously with
   monkeys? Do they have the experience and technical
   training to perform the necessary surgery skillfully?
7. Is Dr. Jones' laboratory adequately equipped for this
   project?
8. Is the institution with which Dr. Jones is affiliated
   registered under the Animal Welfare Act?
9. Is the institution with which Dr. Jones is affiliated
   accredited by AAALAC, or is there an equivalent institutional program of standards maintenance that has been
   accepted by NIH?
10. Does Dr. Jones' institution have a mechanism for evalu-
    ating the humane treatment of animals?

11. What is the basis for Dr. Jones' assurance that the animals would receive adequate veterinary care throughout the study?
12. Has Dr. Jones examined alternative possibilities to the restraint system he proposes to use?
13. What is the evidence that monkeys can be maintained adequately in restraint chairs for such long periods of time?

I think that I know what Dr. Jones' responses to these questions would be; but I propose not to say any more until later, when it may be appropriate to indicate how I would resolve the case.

I hope this brief introduction will have provided sufficient background information to enable each of you now to share your views with the rest of us on the philosophical, ethical, and scientific issues that this case raises. Do the ends justify the means? Is the use of these monkeys appropriate in this instance? Is society correct in placing human interests first? I wish us all a fruitful and rewarding discussion.

Journal Articles:

Dewey J (Sept 1926). The ethics of animal experimentation. Atlantic Monthly.
Shuster S (1978). In ignorance arrayed. Review of "Alternatives to Animal Experiments." Br Med J 1:1541-1542.

Books:

"Guide for the Care and Use of Laboratory Animals" (1978). DHEW Pub No (NIH) 78-23. Revised. 70 pp.
"National Institutes of Health Policy on Humane Care and Use of Animals" (1979). PHS Manual. Chapters 1-43.
Singer P (1975). "Animal Liberation." New York: Random House. 307 pp.
Visscher M (1975). "Ethical Constraints and Imperatives in Medical Research." Springfield, Ill.: CC Thomas. 116 pp.

DISCUSSION SUMMARY: ANIMAL RIGHTS AND ANIMAL EXPERIMENTATION

Marc D. Basson

Director, CEHM
University of Michigan
Ann Arbor, Michigan

Three-fourths of the discussants were willing to approve
the proposed experiment on the basis of the information given
in the case and assumed satisfactory answers to the questions
Bennett Cohen raised in his presentation. One-fourth objected
to the study.

Those who approved of the study generally did so on
utilitarian grounds. They found Regan's theories of animal
rights unconvincing and justified their votes by the potential
good the study could do for other humans, and their ignorance
of any other way in which the relevant knowledge could be
obtained. Many specified that their approval was contingent
on proof that the monkeys would be adequately cared for and
that the study could not be made less painful.

Discussants refusing to approve the experiments, on the
other hand, typically accepted Regan's claim that animals
had rights or at least believed that these monkeys did.
Several argued that while rats might not be sufficiently
intelligent to have rights, chimpanzees certainly did, alluding
to the work that has been done with teaching monkeys American
Sign Language and "Yerkish". One compared the animals in the
study favorably with human neonates. Others attacked the
claim that this experiment was really necessary to promote
even human happiness. Some argued that the goal of preventing
morbidity from myocardial infarctions could be better achieved
by making humans bear the burden of avoiding cigarettes and
high cholesterol foods. Others pointed out that even if this
experiment were essential for decreasing infarct-associated
morbidity, there were still other ways in which human welfare

could be improved significantly without animal experimentation (e.g., better public health education, increasing our
agricultural knowledge to combat world hunger).

Rights and Responsibilities in Modern Medicine: The Second
Volume in a Series on Ethics, Humanism, and Medicine: 95–97
© 1981 Alan R. Liss, Inc.,150 Fifth Avenue, New York, NY 10011

INTRODUCTION: INFORMED CONSENT IN MEDICAL TREATMENT

Doreen Ganos
Director for Publicity and Registration, CEHM
University of Michigan
Ann Arbor, Michigan

Informed consent has become important in medical ethics
since the consumer's rights and other movements have increased
support of paternalistic medicine. It has traditionally been
held that a consent must be voluntary, competent, and informed to be valid. Each of these requirements, however, raises
a number of questions whose answers are not so clear. For
example, what type and degree of coercion, if any, is
acceptable in a "voluntary" choice? What exactly are the
criteria for competency? Does the mere provision of information fulfill one's obligation to inform, or must one
make sure that the information is understood? How much
information is necessary and to what degree must it be
understood?

Though these questions are not unique to medicine, the
medical setting gives them special meaning. When the body
is sick, the mind also suffers. Normal adults, when ill,
tend to regress psychologically, some to an almost childlike
state, and are dependent upon their doctor, whom they usually
view as a parental authority figure. Thus, the doctor-
patient relationship unavoidably provides for a great deal
of coercive power on the physician's side. To what degree
does this power affect the "voluntariness" of the patient's
decision? Furthermore, even in minor illnesses, concentration
and thought processes are impaired by physical and emotional
discomfort. In more severe illnesses, such stress can combine with the direct actions of disease and the side effects
of therapy to seriously impair an otherwise competent person's
ability to think. The case presented for discussion, which
describes a patient whose anxiety, illness, and medication

have made her blind, periodically confused, and suicidally depressed, is a good example of this. At what point should such a patient, who has already been robbed of much of her autonomy by her illness, have the rest stripped from her by being declared incompetent?

The problem of mental impairment is also crucial for the criterion of information. Medicine is such an enormous and complex field that physicians spend years learning small parts of it. How, then, can a patient, impaired by the ravages of disease, be made to understand the risks and benefits of a proposed treatment? Furthermore, how common must a possible complication be to necessitate disclosure (especially since increasing the information provided also increases the patient's anxiety and impairs his comprehension)?

A. Edward Doudera, an attorney with special expertise in the relationship between medicine and the law, explores the legal implications of informed consent. (He concentrates on questions of disclosure and competency since the voluntary nature of a consent would have to be flagrantly violated to be challenged in court.) After explaining that physicians have a positive duty to inform the patient of all relevant facts, with failure to do so considered grounds for a malpractice suit on the basis of negligence, Doudera outlines the kinds of information courts and legislatures have generally considered relevant and some of the standards they have used to measure adequacy of disclosure. He also states that emergencies and therapeutic privilege (withholding relevant data when disclosure of the information would upset the patient so much that he would be unable to effectively weigh the risks of refusing treatment) are considered legal exceptions to the consent requirement, although some argue against the latter on ethical grounds. Lastly, Doudera explains the legal concept of competency, cautioning that the irrationality of a patient's decision does not permit the doctor to declare the patient incompetent as that is for the courts to decide.

Faith Fitzgerald, on the other hand, approaches this issue from a clinician's point of view, and explores ethical rather than legal duties. She emphasizes two primary considerations: the question of understanding and the question of harm. In assessing the question of understanding, Dr. Fitzgerald cites one study (Robinson and Merav, 1976) which indicates that comprehension may be a problem even for

patients whose cognitive functions appear unimpaired.
However, though the study is quite persuasive, it is far
from conclusive, and more recently a similarly designed
study (Woodward, 1979) failed to reach the same conclusions.

Dr. Fitzgerald then takes up the question of harm. She
stresses that disclosure can harm patients not only by increasing their fear and/or depression even to the point of
treatment refusal, but also (as placebo experiments have
shown) by increasing the probability of their developing
one of the complications about which they have been told.
Thus, Fitzgerald defends a somewhat more broadly-defined
therapeutic privilege than Doudera. She then uses this
therapeutic privilege to resolve the ethical conflict between the obligation to impart "full information" and the
duty to do no harm, both prima facie ethical duties for the
physician.

REFERENCES

Robinson G. Merav A (1976). Informed consent: Recall by
    patients tested postoperatively. Ann Thoracic Surg
    22:209.
Woodward W E (1979). Informed consent of volunteers: A
    direct measure of comprehension and retention of
    information. Clinical Research 27:248.

Rights and Responsibilities in Modern Medicine: The Second Volume in a Series on Ethics, Humanism, and Medicine: 99—100
© 1981 Alan R. Liss, Inc., 150 Fifth Avenue, New York, NY 10011

INFORMED CONSENT IN MEDICAL TREATMENT:
HOW MUCH SHOULD THE PATIENT BE TOLD?

Case for Discussion

An 84 year old woman went nearly blind because of an
inflammatory blood vessel disease. She had been active both
physically and mentally for all of her years, swimming at
least two laps a day and reading voraciously. In order to
prevent further diminution of sight, she was placed on high
dose Cortisone. Within the month after her **precipitous**
blindness, she became profoundly depressed. She lost
interest in politics, reading, and her family. She became
periodically confused, claiming not to recognize her
children. She expressed the desire to curl up and die, and
repeatedly asked to be killed. She was admitted to the
Neuropsychiatric Institute.

Because of her unstable cardiovascular status, and the
severity of her suicidal ideas, it was felt that the
psychotropic drugs would either be dangerous (from the point
of view of their side effects) or take too long to have an
effect. Electroconvulsive (shock) therapy would be the
quickest therapy.

Risks of ECT included irregular rhythms of her heart,
potential bone damage from convulsion, and further brain
damage.

The questions to be asked were:

1. Could this woman, with known brain disease and
periods of confusion, understand the potential risks and
benefits of therapy sufficiently to give informed consent?

2.   If this woman is deemed capable of giving
informed consent during the periods in which her mental status is as it was prior to her disease, how much should she
be told about the risks of ECT?

3.   Since one of the known effects of electroconvulsive
therapy is loss of memory, would an informed consent given
at the initiation of therapy hold throughout the course?
Would we have to repeat the information, memory of which
could be ablated by the therapy itself, before each
successive treatment?

Prepared by Faith T. Fitzgerald

Rights and Responsibilities in Modern Medicine: The Second
Volume in a Series on Ethics, Humanism, and Medicine: 101–111
© 1981 Alan R. Liss, Inc., 150 Fifth Avenue, New York, NY 10011

INFORMED CONSENT: HOW MUCH SHOULD THE PATIENT KNOW?

A. Edward Doudera, J.D.

Executive Director, American Society of Law &
     Medicine
Boston, Massachusetts

In the case to be discussed, an 84 year old woman, who
was previously quite active, both mentally and physically,
loses her sight due to a blood vessel disease. She is treated
with Cortisone, and about a month later becomes quite depressed:
losing interest in politics, not "recognizing" her children,
and expressing the view that she wants to die. In the facts
supplied, she has been admitted to the Neuropsychiatric Institute -- it is unclear, however, whether it was her decision
or that of her children. In order not to complicate the situation more than is necessary, we'll assume the patient sought
hospitalization and treatment on her own. Her physicians have
examined her and determined that electro-convulsive therapy
[ECT] is the indicated medical treatment, but before they can
proceed, they need the patient's consent. There are two legal
issues presented: 1) what is informed consent and what are
its essential elements, and 2) is this individual capable or
competent to give an informed consent. The problem is, simply,
that if the patient is not competent to give her consent or if
the information disclosed by the physician was insufficient,
no valid consent exists and the physician, or hospital, would
be liable.

WHY DO WE NEED INFORMED CONSENT?

The doctrine of informed consent is based upon a fundamental Anglo-American legal theory -- that the unprivileged,
unauthorized, intentional touching of a person by another is a
"battery," a crime at common law. The first function of the
doctrine is, therefore, to preserve the integrity of each

person's own body. As such, medical or surgical procedures
performed without the consent of the patient constitute
legal battery and give rise to a civil cause of action for
damages. The consent is the patient's authorization to the
doctor to do the procedures and protects the physician from
liability.

The first reported case which required the patient's[1]
consent to medical treatment is an English case from 1767.
The most frequently cited American case is one from 1914 where
Justice Cardozo stated: "Every human being of adult years
and sound mind has a right to determine what shall be done
with his own body; and a surgeon who performs an operation
without his patient's consent commits an assault." [2]

Today, however, the legal authority behind the doctrine
of informed consent has generally moved away from this "battery" foundation and is founded in the constitutionally protected right of privacy which has been held to extend to
unwanted infringements upon the bodily integrity of patients.[3]
This trend away from "battery" is highlighted in the opinion
of the Massachusetts Supreme Judicial Court In the Matter of
Earle Spring,[4] where the court noted that the traditional
legal concept of battery did not fit neatly within the factual
realities of the doctor-patient relationship, especially when
we consider the withdrawal of medical treatment from an incompetent patient. The re-definition of the legal basis for
informed consent has strengthened the patient's right to full
and complete information concerning proposed medical procedures or treatments. Further, many states have enacted specific statutes which address this issue: For example, the
Michigan Public Health Code includes a Patient's Statement of
Rights which affirms the "right of an adult, competent patient
to be inviolate in his person and to accept medical care or
treatment only with his or her informed consent."[5]

Under this theory, the physician has an affirmative duty
to the patient to disclose all relevant and material facts,
including the risks of treatment. Failure to disclose completely is treated as negligence.[6] This obligation is created by the doctor-patient relationship and gives rise to a
second function of informed consent -- to encourage rational
medical decision-making. The doctrine of informed consent can
be viewed as a guardian of individualism in the medical context; it protects the patient's right of self-determination in
medical matters as well as the patient's right to privacy.[7]

WHAT IS INFORMED CONSENT?

Informed consent has been defined in a variety of ways, most simply as: A free decision based upon adequate information. George Annas has described the doctrine as follows:

> A physician may not treat a patient until he has explained to the patient the risk and material facts concerning the treatment and its alternatives, including nontreatment, and has secured the patient's competent, voluntary, and understanding consent to proceed.[8]

An "informed consent" has two distinct elements: 1) disclosure, and 2) awareness and assent. Awareness and assent (or competency) affect the consent portion; disclosure addresses the informed component. The essential elements that must be disclosed to a patient are:
1) the nature and purpose of the proposed procedures
2) the likelihood of success
3) the hazards of the procedure, and
4) alternative treatments, including nontreatment.[9]

An informed consent can be both oral and written. In practice, much of the discussion concerning "informed consent" focusses upon the consent form and not the essentials of the consent itself. Physicians often ignore the difference between substance (the actual conversation between physician and patient concerning what the physician intends to do and why, what the alternatives are, and what the probabilities of success and the risks may be) and form (the permission slip that many hospitals require to be signed as evidence of consent.) The written consent form is only a piece of evidence that documents the transaction between doctor and patient which gave rise to the patient consenting to the recommended treatment. Although many studies have attempted to challenge the validity of informed consent,[10] Society has clearly adopted the doctrine. Physicians will never (nor should they) be immune to litigation brought by patients who reject, forget, misinterpret, or deny their efforts to inform. However, by attempting to improve the communication process and the readability of consent forms, and by accepting the education of the patient through the process of consent as a worthwhile therapeutic goal, physicians can assure that the processes of informed consent are fulfilled.

IS IT IMPORTANT?

It is important to remember that lack of informed consent is a separate tort and that liability can attach absent any findings of negligence or malpractice. For example, in 1977, a one million dollar verdict was given to a paralyzed patient solely on the basis of lack of informed consent. In this case, the physician failed to disclose the risk of paralysis inherent to the aortic surgery being recommended. The physician testified that the procedure was strongly indicated by the patient's case history, that he feared the patient would reject the surgery if its inherent risk of paralysis was disclosed, and that he decided, therefore, not to disclose the risk.[11] The jury was not impressed and found for the patient.

THE EXTENT OF DISCLOSURE, OR DID THE PATIENT KNOW ENOUGH?

One of the most perplexing questions asked by physicians is: How much must I disclose and explain to a patient? Essentially, there are three tests used by courts in determining the adequacy of the disclosure made by a physician seeking a patient's consent:

1) Objective or professional standard test -- where the the physician's obligation is to provide the patient with information similar to that provided by other physicians doing similar procedures. In a lawsuit, the plaintiff/patient would have to show that the physician did not disclose some risk or alternative treatment that his colleagues generally told their patients. This standard, first articulated in 1960 in Natanson v. Kline,[12] is still the majority rule.

2) The subjective test, which is the least followed, relies upon the patient's understanding of the explanation of the risks and probable consequences. If the patient did not understand the real risks of the procedure, there was no consent given.

3) The third, and future trend, was adopted in Canterbury v. Spence,[13] where the court discarded the "professional standard" for one imposed by law, and stated that whether the physician's disclosure was reasonable, and therefore legally sufficient, depends on what the physician knows, or should know, to be the patient's need for information. If a risk or danger of the proposed treat-

ment could be material to the patient's decision to accept or reject the treatment, it must
be disclosed. Similarly, in Cobbs v. Grant, 14
the California court stated that the duty to
disclose was measured by whatever information
a reasonable patient finds material to making
his decision. The court stated that when a
given procedure inherently involves a known
risk of death or serious bodily harm, the
physician has a duty to disclose the potential
of death or of serious harm and to explain in
lay terms the complications that might occur.

In a lawsuit, the plaintiff has the burden of proving
the materiality of the undisclosed risk; a question which
turns on the "seriousness of the consequences, the probability
of occurence, and the feasibility of alternatives."15 One case
which attempted to explain "material" versus "non-material"
risks held that a risk was insignificant if its probability
of occurence ranged from 3/4 of one percent to zero percent. 16

One of the newer approaches to the problem of disclosure
is that taken by the Texas legislature. 17 Under 1977 legislation, a Medical Disclosure Panel -- which consists of 6
doctors and 3 lawyers -- is charged with spelling out which
risks a physician must disclose to a patient and which procedures require no disclosure at all. According to the Houston
surgeon who chairs the panel, the law is premised upon the
idea that there is no such thing as informed consent. He
cites three reasons:
   a) the infinite number of potential risks,
   b) the patient's inability to grasp the information
      relayed by the physician, and
   c) the emotionally charged medical situation itself.
The panel is simply deciding whether a procedure is on list A
or list B; whether it requires or does not require disclosure
of inherent risks. The question supposedly asked is:
      Whether knowing about the inherent hazards
      of a procedure would deter a reasonable and
      prudent person from consenting to it.
For procedures included in list A -- those that require disclosure -- the panel is specifying what risks must be disclosed.
Presently, no one procedure has been finalized.

The law would give statutory protection to physicians who
utilized the approved consent form which would itemize the

risks in the procedure. The physician would have no obligation to disclose any other risks. Whether this approach is
successful, only time will tell.

WHEN NOT TO DISCLOSE

There are exceptions to the requirement of informed consent -- for example, emergencies, where it is implied that if
the injured/unconscious person could have consented, he would
have consented to procedures intended to save him or bring him
to a stable or cognizant state. The courts have also recognized a "therapeutic privilege" for physicians to withhold
otherwise material information in situations where the facts
reasonably demonstrate that disclosure would so seriously upset the patient that he or she would not be able to weigh the
risks of refusing to undergo the recommended treatment.[18] We
get legally effective, but by no means informed, consent.
Some commentators have stated that the exception must be accompanied by a presumption that all patients are capable of
dealing with complete disclosure,[19] thereby placing the burden
upon physicians to defend non-disclosure.

Robert Veatch, previously from the Hastings Center, recently expressed the view that if we are to accord patients
their right of self-determination in medical decisions and
their right of bodily integrity, then the doctrine of therapeutic privilege is not ethically defendable. Patients, he
contends, must be told the truth concerning their medical
condition. Physicians are consultants to patients, and patients, not physicians, must finally decide upon their own best
interests.

Lastly, it must be noted that physicians have no obligation to disclose any risk or otherwise material facts where
a competent patient explicitly or knowingly waives his right
to be so advised.

COMPETENCY AND THE RIGHTS OF INCOMPETENT PATIENTS

In obtaining a valid consent, it is essential that the
patient must be competent to understand the risks, benefits
and alternatives of the proposed treatment, and the issue of
competency is determined as of the time the consent is obtained.
The patient asked to consent must normally be an adult who

comprehends the nature and gravity of a proposed procedure.
In assessing competency, it is generally appropriate to consider whether the patient has the ability to manage his affairs with ordinary or reasonable prudence, has demonstrated
rational understanding or intellectual comprehension, is capable of making a full deliberation of matters presented to
him, has the mental capacity to make choices, or has the substantial capacity to understand and appreciate the nature and
the consequences of a specified matter.[20]

A patient who is intoxicated or drugged may not be able
to give a valid informed consent. For example, the consent
of a competent person could be invalidated if it could be
shown that the person was on medications which affected the
essentials of the consent process -- voluntariness, competency,
and knowledge of the relevant facts.[21]

It is essential that we recognize that incompetent patients are entitled to the same rights afforded competent
patients. The issue, rather, is how best to give effect to
these rights.

Historically, mental patients have not been afforded
rights to consent to medical treatment. The state used its
power to act as a guardian for the committed, and consented
to medical or psychiatric care where appropriate, presumably
acting in the patient's best interest. This denial of informed consent rights was based on notions of competency and
contractual validity. Just as a lunatic could not be held to
a contract, neither could he give legally effective consent
to medical treatment.[22] However, significant changes have
occurred in recent years. Many courts have determined that
the fact of institutionalization does not in and of itself
create a status of incompetency or give rise to a presumption
of inability to manage one's affairs.[23] Rather, individualized
determinations of one's ability to make decisions concerning
specific aspects of one's own affairs are being required.

Recently, federal district courts in Massachusetts and
New Jersey have ruled that institutionalized mental patients
have a constitutional right to refuse treatment, including medication and seclusion.[24] The decision affirms the view that
individuals do not lose their rights to privacy and to free
expression merely by being confined in a mental institution.
To quote the Rogers opinion:
            The fact that mind control takes place

> in a mental institution in the form of
> medically sound treatment of mental disease
> is not, itself, an extraordinary circum-
> stance warranting an unsanctioned intrusion
> on the integrity of a human being.

Exceptions would be allowed, the court noted, but only in
situations where "extreme violence, personal injury, or attempted suicide" were presented. (It should be noted that
refusing treatment cannot be equated with suicide since the
patient is not responsible for his medical condition -- the
result of which is death).

When dealing with an incompetent individual it is necessary to have a guardian appointed to make decisions where the
patient would otherwise have a right of informed consent.[25]
When physicians are uncertain about a patient's competency,
they would be wise to get a guardian appointed, at least for
the specific purpose of consenting to treatment, rather than
risk liability should the patient later be found incompetent
and the treatment rendered, therefore, an assault. However,
recognize here too, that a real medical emergency will remove
the obligation to get consent from the patient, be he competent or incompetent.

One problem when dealing with patients who are suspected
of being incompetent is that physicians tend to think patients
"competent" so long as they follow the suggested procedures.
However, when the patient rejects their advice, the same patient is considered being "incompetent." For example, in a
case where a woman refused to consent to the amputation of her
leg, her competence to consent was not questioned until she
rejected the medical advice of her physician. But as the court
stated:

> the irrationality of her decision does
> not justify a conclusion that [she] is
> incompetent in the legal sense. The law
> protects her right to make her own decision
> to accept or reject treatment, whether that
> decision is wise or unwise.[26]

Recent cases in Massachusetts and New Jersey, among others,
indicate that it is the courts, however, not the medical profession, who decide who is or is not competent. Clearly, testimony by psychiatrists and others is taken, but the court
ultimately decides. Thus, in the New Jersey case, a 72 year
old man refused to consent to the amputation of his gangre-

nous leg. The doctors went to court to have him declared incompetent and to have a guardian appointed to consent to the
treatment. At the hearing, the psychiatric testimony was
split concerning competency and the judge actually visited the
patient in the hospital before finding the patient competent.
The court went on to hold that the right of privacy permits
a patient to decline treatment where an extensive bodily inva-
sion is involved.[27] Such a right exists for all patients and
the opportunity to exercise it must be respected by all health
care providers.

CONCLUSION

Returning to the case discussed in the first paragraph
of this article, the question with which we are faced is:
> Whether this patient is competent and
> capable of understanding the proposed
> medical intervention?

If she is, then the law requires the disclosure to her of
all material information and permits her to reject the treatment. We can discuss the extent of disclosure, but its need
is clear.

If she is believed to be incompetent, or that she will
become incompetent during the course of the proposed treatment, her rights still apply, and it is necessary to have a
guardian appointed for the purpose of exercising her rights.

It would be totally illegal and unethical for a physician
to decide what is "best" for the patient and to proceed with
the planned course of treatment without the consent of the
patient or her guardian if incompetency has been properly
adjudicated. The fact that the patient ultimately survives
does not legitimize the physician's action, it simply reduces
the changes that the physician will be sued for his or her
behavior.

REFERENCES

1. Slater v. Baker & Stapleton, 95 Eng. Rep. 860 (K.B.
1767).
2. Schloendorff v. Society of New York Hospital, 105 N.E.
92, 93 (NY 1914).

3. <u>In Matter of Quinlan</u>, 355 A.2d 647 (N.J. 1976);
<u>Superintendent of Belchertown State School</u> v. <u>Saikewicz</u>, 370
N.E. 2d 417 (Mass. 1977). Both Quinlan and Saikewicz deal
with the question of withholding life-supporting procedures
from an incompetent individual and both affirm the individual's constitutional right of privacy to reject even life-
saving treatment. The cases recognize four state interests
that could combine to outweigh the right of the individual to
exercise this right: interest in the preservation of life;
the prevention of suicide; the need to protect innocent third
parties; and the ethical integrity of the medical profession.
4. <u>In the Matter of Earle N. Spring</u>
5. MCC §333.20201
6. The first case to so hold was <u>Salgo</u> v. <u>Leland Stanford Jr., University Board of Trustees</u>, 154 Cal. App. 2d 560,
317 P.2d 170 (Dist. Ct. of App. 1957).
7. Mersel A, (1979). The exceptions to the informed
consent doctrine: striking a balance between competing values
in medical decision-making. Wisconsin Law Review: 413.
8. Annas GA (1975). "Rights of Hospital Patients."
New York: Avon Books, p. 57.
9. Some writers want even more disclosed: diagnosis,
choice of treatment; alternative treatments including no
treatment at all; specific methods to be used in the course
of treatment; potential risks; side-effects and benefits of
treatment; future risks; expected pain and discomfort; and
prognosis. [(1970). **Restructuring informed consent: legal
therapy for the doctor-patient** relationship. Yale Law Journal:
79:1533.]
10. <u>See</u>, e.g., Laforet EG (1976). The fiction of informed
consent. J. Am. Medical Association 235:1579-85; Cassileth
BR, <u>et al</u>., Informed consent: why are its goals imperfectly
realized?. New England J of Medicine 302(16):896-900 (Ap 7,
1980); Grundner TM (Ap 17, 1980). On the readability of surgical consent forms. New England J of Medicine 302(16):900-
02.
11. <u>Jones</u> v. <u>Regents of the University of California</u>,
Super Ct., San Francisco Co., Calif. 1977.
12. 186 Kan. 383, 350 P.2d 1093 (1960).
13. 464 F.2d 722 (D.C. Cir. 1972).
14. 8 Ca. 3d 229, 502 P.2d 1 (1972).
15. <u>Lambert</u> v. <u>Park</u>, 597 F.2d 236 (10th Cir. 1979).
16. <u>Mason</u> v. <u>Ellsworth</u>, 474 P.2d 909 (Wash. App. 1970).
17. Curran WJ(1979). Informed consent, Texas style: disclosure and nondisclosure by regulation. New England J of
Medicine 300(9):482.

18. Cobbs v. Grant, 8 Cal. 2d 229, 502 P.2d 1 (1972); Natanson v. Kline, 186 Kan. 393, 350 P.2d 1093 (1960); Roberts v. Wood, 206 F Supp 579 (S.D. Ala. 1962); Nishi v. Hartwell, 52 Haw. 188, 473 P.2d 116 (1970); Ball v. Mallinkrodt Chem. Works, 53 Tenn. App. 218, 381 S.W.2d 536 (tenn Ct. App. 1964).

19. Annas GA (1975). "The Rights of Hospital Patients." New York: Avon Books, p. 62.

20. "Consent Handbook."(1977). Washington, D.C.: American Association on Mental Deficiency, p. 7.

21. Demers v. Gerety, 515 P.2d 645 (N.M.Ct. App. 1973) (Patient given sleeping pill and awakened in middle of night to sign consent form; consent invalidated because patient had no recollection thereof).

22. See, e.g., Dexter v. Hall, 82 US (15 Wall.) 9 (1872).

23. Vecchoine v. Wohlgemuth, 377 F.Supp. 1367 (E.D.Pa. 1974).

24. Rogers v. Okin, 478 F. Supp. 134 (D. Mass. 1979); Rennie v. Klein, 476 F. Supp. 1294 (N.J. 1979).

25. Matter of Schiller, 372 A.2d 360 (N.J. Super 1977).

26. Lane v. Candura, 376 N.E. 2d 1232 (Mass. App. 1978).

27. Matter of Robert Quackenbush, An Alleged Incompetent, 383 A. 2d 785 (Morris Co. Ct., N.J. 1978).

Rights and Responsibilities in Modern Medicine: The Second
Volume in a Series on Ethics, Humanism, and Medicine: 113–121
© 1981 Alan R. Liss, Inc., 150 Fifth Avenue, New York, NY 10011

INFORMED CONSENT

Faith T. Fitzgerald, M.D.

University of Michigan Medical Center

Ann Arbor, Michigan   48109

I'd like to correct the title given me in the schedule
of speakers. I am not the Director of Inpatient Programming,
which smacks of a computerized, robotized futurism in which
I program inpatients. I am, rather, Director of Inpatient
Programs i.e. clinical and teaching activities which occur
on the Inpatient Internal Medicine Wards at University
Hospital, Ann Arbor. Maybe it was in honor of the topic
today – informed consent – that a Freudian slip was made.
Clearly, the recent flurry of legal and ethical inquiry
into questions of informed consent suggests that somebody
out there suspects physicianry of being inclined to
program their patients rather then to inform them.

Examination of the issues of informed consent is an
everyday activity for me. As a clinician, I want the
best for my patients; as an administrator, I am involved
in setting the rules which supposedly govern other
physicians in this hospital in their relationship with
patients; and, most importantly, as a teacher, I am
responsible for "setting the good example", for being
the pattern upon which students mold their behavior in
dealings with their future patients.

It is with the question of ethics, of right and wrong,
of morality in fact, that I choose to wrestle today, leaving
the still evolving questions of law to the more learned
Mr. Doudera. And since I am a clinician and an internist
(rather than an investigator or pediatrician), I'll fix
specifically on the problems that come up in the everyday
practice of adult medicine rather then spend time on the

ethical problems of informed consent in experimentation or in children.

The World Medical Association Declaration of 1964 stated "The doctor should obtain the patient's freely given consent after the patient has been given full information." (Ludlam, J 1978) This is a logical derivative of Judge Cardozo's belief of 50 years before, that "Every human being of adult years and sound mind has a right to determine what shall be done with his own body." (Dellinger, A.M. and Warren D.G. 1972) Agreeing fully with these principles, the two major problems I encounter most frequently in my daily practice are:

1. The question of understanding: Can an individual patient, altered by disease, emotional stress, or intellectual impairment, truly assimilate, assess, and judge "full information"?

2. The question of harm: Are there circumstances in which, by imparting "full information", I frighten or disturb my patient to such a degree that they, through fear or depression, refuse essential therapy or - if they allow it - suffer more complications from it because of anxiety and stress?

Both of these questions are touched upon in the patient represented in the case I've given you for today's discussion: A woman, depressed and periodically confused, is offered a therapy which - though it may make her dramatically better - may also confuse her further and could potentially kill her.

A delightful eighty-four year old woman, vigorous and active (she used to swim two laps a day) was afflicted with a disease causing inflammation of the blood vessels of the brain and the eye. The inflammation caused swelling, the swelling led to a decrease in blood flow, and that decrease in blood flow to her brain caused confusional episodes, and to her eyes blindness. So from an alert, productive woman she within several weeks turned into a periodically confused, sensorially deprived, dependent woman.

The therapy for this form of vascular inflammation is

very high dose cortisone. Cortisone in high doses can
cause emotional changes, leading to lability of mood,
depression, and several other complications.

After about two months of her progressive blindess,
episodic confusion, and probably some of the depressive
effects of the cortisone, she grew profoundly depressed.
She curled up into a ball and would say nothing but "I
want to die", and then "I am dead". She had literally
declared herself dead.

I consulted a psychiatrist. We agreed that there were
three ways of handling this from a therapeutic standpoint:

1) The woman was active and productive, and her
chances for recovery from her blindness were unknown. She's
quite appropriately depressed, and she's made a thoroughly
rational decision to die. Let's leave her alone.

2) We may put her on phenothiazines - Thorazine,
Stelazine, Mellaril - what have you. Any of the psycho-
therapeutic drugs, however, have attendant risks of major
complications, including irregular rhythms of the heart,
neurologic defects, and sudden death.

3) Or, we can consider shock therapy: Apply
electricity across her brain and, in some circumstances,
this will give a remarkable recovery. But it also has
risks - seizures, amongst other things - and an eighty-four
year old woman could break bones during a fit, further
immobilizing her. And one of the ways shock therapy may
work in depression is by ablating recent memory, and she
is already profoundly depressed by her loss of memory. I
may, by my therapy, confuse her further.

So as I walk to her room, I know she's lying there
saying "I am dead", and that I must try to get her
informed consent to one of these three alternatives.

An interesting problem, and a very real one. I'll
tell you how it came out when you've decided what you would
do.

THE QUESTION OF UNDERSTANDING:

Let's open with this question, since it obviously obtains in my patient. Am I, at any point in time, speaking to her in a period of lucidity or one of confusion, since she alternates so? Can she understand what I am trying to tell her? Let us accept that every adult patient of sound mind has the right to know the nature of their illness, the proposed treatment, the physician's experience with that treatment, the kind and amount of anticipated pain, the likely benefits of treatment, alternatives to the proposed treatment, and the prognosis.

Let us even hypothesize that all physicians agree to this (and they seem not to: In a handbook to clinical procedures for medical students written by a surgeon, I find the following quote: "...the request for permission should be presented to the patient in such a way that he feels he has no option to refuse. By that, I mean that it is best to be firm and authoritative, stressing that no other course is possible. Such an approach, if presented in a pleasant manner, will do much to gain the patient's cooperation and prevent refusal...despite all efforts to the contrary, there will still be a few patients who defy rational management and refuse to cooperate. Restraint is occasionally necessary for the confused and irrational adult. If general obstinacy or adamant refusal prevents the completion of a procedure...(don't) waste further time." (Fisher, JC 1977) None of this "informed consent" Nonsense for him, obviously.) But let's assume I want to do the right thing. I want my patient, whose life it is, to decide what she wants to do with it. But she's suicidally depressed, and periodically confused. Can I get informed consent? Given her periods of confusion, we might well say that the best thing to do is to go to someone else, her lineal kin who are responsible agents. But she's periodically not confused and had always been fiercely independent of her children. Can I force her to abrogate her adulthood to them during the intervals of her lucidity?

A striking study that I have referenced for you shows that the question is a real one even in less blatant settings. (Robinson, G and Merav A 1976) Drs. Robinson and Merav carefully documented by tape recording their complete informed consent interviews with 20 preoperative patients. Four to six months later, they found the the vast majority of these patients were unable to remember, not only the specifics of what had been discussed, but even that the discussion had taken place at all. Yet at the time of the informed consent, all indices were that each of the twenty gave a truly informed consent to their operations. How do we know, ever, that our patient's consent is understood? How long will they understand to what they have assented?

Drs. Robinson and Merav have fulfilled the letter of the law regarding informed consent - but can I, knowing of their study, be comfortable once I've gone through a lucid and careful explanation to my patient, and my patient responded with seeming understanding, that I have discharged my ethical obligation? It shouldn't have surprised me: It takes me weeks to years to instill principles of diagnosis, alternative therapy, risk and prognosis into medical students (who are not terribly emotionally involved) and they forget! How shall I expect my patients to understand these same principles, particularly as they apply in emotionally charged situations, after one or two tries at explanation. This is true even in patients whom all of us would accept as fully rational adults, and how much more true it might be in those who's cognitive function - as in my lady presented today - has been altered by disease or therapy. Well, one can but try - but do we? This brings up:

THE QUESTION OF HARM:

In my patient, severely depressed by her debility from her blindness, shall I not depress her further by acknowledging that she might suffer yet more debility from the therapy I propose?

It is a common argument by physicians, that they might scare their patients with the truth. In Oken's study (Oken 1961) of more than 200 physicians, nearly nine out of ten revealed that they do not tell a patient that the diagnosis is cancer. The reason given by the majority of doctors for their silence was that they might, by telling, rob their patients of sustaining hope. Things have changed some since 1961. For one thing, 3 surveys of cancer patients show 80% or more are glad to have been told their diagnosis. Still, though I believe doctors are more informative now than they were 18 years ago, many

hold on to the conviction that they might hurt their
patients with full disclosure.

I spoke to an eminent cardiologist in this city a
few days ago. I said, "What do you do when a patient
comes in for a cardiac catheterization, and they are
obviously concerned by their symptoms of chest pain and
palpitations, and fearful of sudden death? Do you fully
explain to such a patient that the complications of the
cardiac catheterization might include sudden death?"
He said, "Well...I don't always do that. If I tell them
such a thing, and they are highly anxious already, they
may grow more anxious yet. And one of the features of
great anxiety is the release of adrenalin into the
bloodstream, and a more rapid heartbeat in consequence of
that. That increase in rate, and sometimes irregularity
of rhythm from the adrenalin may actually increase their
chance of sudden death. So by revealing to the patient
what the complications might be, I might actually pre-
cipitate them. I might cause a problem that otherwise
would not have occured."

It is assuredly the case that there are frightening
facts and highly emotional patients who might be devis-
tated, by these facts. What is best is not always clear.
What is necessary, I think, is that physicians continually
examine their motives for witholding information from the
patient. I should be certain, when I do, that my action
is based on what is best for the patient rather than
what is convenient - either emotionally or physically -
for me.

The original meaning of the word "doctor", i.e.
teacher, was well chosen. My job is to take the information that the patient gives me by history and physical
examination, to structure it according to my knowledge
and experience into some logical explanations, and
redeliver these in an understandable way back to the
patient along with several options as to what to do about
it. It is the patient's job to decide amongst those
options, as to which - if any - he or she shall exercise.

But for both of us, physician and patient, the job
isn't always going to be easy.

Q. What if the patient says, "Doctor - you make the

choice?"

A. What I generally do is proceed along with an
explanation anyhow. I tell them what their options are,
the complications, the probable chances for success and
so on. If then the patient tells me to choose, I
interpret that as asking for my advice. I will then tell
them which of the options seems best to me, which they
may accept as my choice. If they simply lie there and
adamantly refuse to participate in their own care, and
have no relatives to whom I may turn, then I will proceed
in this consentual vacuum to do what I think is right for
them. I must, however, satisfy myself that their refusal
to participate is a real choice on their part, that they
are not doing it because they are afraid of me or too upset
to function at all, or whatever.

Q. What if, in the procedure or therapy you propose,
there is a very real and high risk of death or dying, of
paralysis or some other terrible thing?

A. In that case, we're dealing with a therapeutic
ratio question: Is the chance of benefit from this
procedure or therapy worth the risk of the procedure or
therapy. If there is a great risk that a patient will
come to grief if they suffer the complications of a
procedure or therapy, I must be assured that there is a
very, very great chance that they will be improved by it
if all goes well.

If a single, adult patient of intact reason has chosen
to let me make the decision, I will honor that decision of
theirs as much as any other. I am sometimes discussing a
possible test or drug with a patient in the presence of
the family, and the family begins to interact. On occasion,
the patient will turn to them and say, "Now you people
mean well, but you aren't my doctor. I want Doctor
Fitzgerald to make this decision". That seems to me to be
a valid patient option, to give over as they desire.

In the patient I presented to you today, the actual
events were as follows: I kept asking her, and had the
family asking her, what she wanted us to do. She replied,
for several days, that she was dead. Then, one morning,
she said "Do whatever you like". And, with her family's
consent, I arranged for her to undergo a sequence of

electroshock sessions. After the fourth such session,
she was animated, alert, and conversant and began to
recognize her family, take an interest in ward activities,
and - at this moment - is undergoing plans for discharge
home with a live-in nurse to help her with the affairs of
daily living in which she is still compromised by her
blindness.

Q. If somebody was undergoing a procedure or operation
which had a complication which would be increased if you
were to tell them about it, would you tell them what the
complications were? I thought you said that you wouldn't.

A. I said I didn't know if I would. I don't know
the answer to that question. That would depend upon me,
and that patient, at that point in time and that particular
situation. What I can say is that I cannot categorically
come out and declare that I am going to tell every patient
every thing.

Q. Can you think of examples where there is documented evidence that full disclosure does increase the
risk of complications?

A. Well, only in analogy to placebo drug studies.
Human drug trials often take the form of dividing the
subjects into three groups: Those on no treatment,
placebo, and active pharmacologic agent. All three
groups are informed of the possible risks and complications
of the active agent. It has been found that a number of
those in the placebo group suffer from symptoms suggestive
of the side effects of the active drug.

So far as I know, it's not well documented that you
will hurt somebody - for example the cardiac catheterization
patient - by telling him the truth. Physicians tend to
believe that if a patient is highly agitated and full of
fear, rattling off a list of possible complications to that
patient is not soothing and may agitate them further.

The real question that I would have in that regard is:
Is what the lady in the next bed down says to my patient
worse than the truth, "My grandmother had that test, and
she lost both legs..." And that's so common. I'm
perpetually amazed at the things people tell each other
in their attempts to comfort or be friendly. So I'm

inclined to tell my patients what is true just to protect them from each other and the general misinformation that floats around. But I cannot guarantee that I'd do that for everybody.

REFERENCES

Dellinger AM, Warren D G (1972). Health Law Review
    June: 34.
Fisher JC (1977). "Clinical Procedures." Baltimore:
    Williams and Wilkins Co.
Ludlan J (1978). " Informed Consent." Chicago:
    American Hospital Association.
Oken (1961). What to tell cancer patients. JAMA
    175:1120.
Robinson G, Merav A (1976). Informed consent: Recall
    by patients tested postoperatively. Ann Thoracic
    Surg 22:209.

**Rights and Responsibilities in Modern Medicine: The Second
Volume in a Series on Ethics, Humanism, and Medicine: 123–124
© 1981 Alan R. Liss, Inc., 150 Fifth Avenue, New York, NY 10011**

DISCUSSION SUMMARY: INFORMED CONSENT IN MEDICAL TREATMENT

Doreen Ganos
Director for Publicity and Registration, CEHM
University of Michigan
Ann Arbor, Michigan

All the participants rejected the cynical approach of
the surgeon quoted by Dr. Fitzgerald and upheld the importance of informed consent. Attempting to resolve the
case in question, most of the discussion groups concentrated
on the questions of what constitutes "competency" and how
much must be disclosed to fulfill the requirement of information before consent. A few groups also wrestled with
the effect of electroshock's memory ablation on informed
consent.

After some debate, the participants decided that the
compacity for comprehension and rational choice was essential
for competency. Given this patient's periodic confusion
and the patent irrationality of her statement "I am dead,"
the majority (about 3/4) therefore wished to declare the
woman incompetent. The minority emphasized that the patient
was lucid between her periods of confusion. They argued
that they would prefer to err on the side of autonomy and
wished to accept a properly obtained informed consent
obtained during one of the patient's lucid periods.

Most of the participants agreed that all information
(including risks and alternatives) that could possibly be
deemed relevant must be revealed to the patient if she is
competent. Two of the groups were willing to permit the
withholding of information that might result in harm to
the patient. (One specified that a third party be consulted
before the decision to withhold is made.) However, neither
group indicated that they felt the withholding of information
on the basis of therapeutic privilege to be ethically

justified in this case. Of the groups that considered the relationship between electroshock and the informed consent, about half decided that even if an informed consent were obtained initially, the memory loss associated the ECT would invalidate it. They therefore felt that it would be necessary to obtain new consent after each course of therapy. (They also pointed out the additional knowledge about the nature of ECT which the patient would gain by experience.) However, the rest felt that the initial consent would be valid for the duration unless the patient, while still competent, subsequently opposed continuance of the treatments.

Fifth Conference on
Ethics, Humanism, and Medicine
March 29, 1980

INTRODUCTION TO THE FIFTH CONFERENCE: THE ROLE OF MEDICINE

Marc D. Basson
Director, CEHM
University of Michigan
Ann Arbor, Michigan

Good morning, and welcome to the conference.

If medical ethics is different from any other form of
ethics, it must be because medicine is perceived as a unique
endeavor with special goals and therefore with special
responsibilities incumbent upon its practitioners. Before
we can begin to consider what Dr. X must do in situation Y,
we must first have decided what doctors in general are supposed to be doing. What is medicine all about?

One's first inclination is to say that doctors are
supposed to diagnose and treat disease. This is certainly
at least part of the truth. As we sit here, doctors are
writing prescriptions, making diagnoses and performing surgery. But some of the prescriptions are for Valium rather
than antibiotics. Some of the diagnoses are "anemia
secondary to malnutrition" and "battered child syndrome."
Some of the operations involve cosmetic surgery or abortion.
One patient was to be told this morning that she has un-
resectable cancer. I hope that there is someone there
to listen to her cry.

It is clear that only the broadest definition of disease
can even approach the range of evils which medicine combats.
Perhaps we ought to return to the original etymology and
say that a disease is anything which causes dis-ease in
our patient, whether it be somatic, psychological or societal.
This is an old medical model, dating back when we lacked good
therapy for most biological disorders and the doctor/priest/
father figure/shaman offered as his major therapy supportive

counselling and placebo remedies.

With modern biomedical investigation has come new understanding of the etiology of somatic disorders, so that we have achieved the ability to treat effectively and, perhaps more importantly, to prevent many diseases. We have learned about sanitary precautions and proper nutrition and more recently even about the Type A personality who is more prone to ulcers and myocardial infarctions. One of the most important words in the medicine of the future may be "diathesis," a tendency or predisposition to develop disease because of some condition often invisible without special medical testing.

Because of our new insight into the causes of illness, medicine has undergone an almost Kuhnian paradigm shift in which health is now viewed as an entity in its own right apart from the absence of disease, an entity to be sought and done penance for and in general to be worshipped devoutly by a new sort of medical priesthood and its flock. Type A personalities must be taught to relax. The inactive must be persuaded to jog regularly. Like expensive foreign sports cars, we must keep fine-tuned and smooth-running with periodic checkups and adjustments. It is no longer sufficient to merely function well enough to clunk back and forth to work and the grocery store with an occasional long drive out to the beach.

In 1946, the World Health Organization proposed promoting "health" rather than curing disease as the goal of medicine. In keeping with the old tradition of medical concern with all dis-ease, the WHO defined health as "a state of complete physical, mental and social well-being, and not merely the absence of disease or infirmity." Physicians and philosophers alike have been taking potshots at this definition and the paradigm it symbolizes ever since. They argue that it represents a ridiculous ideal, unattainable and far too inclusive, and hold up for mockery the World Health Organization's more recent goal of "health by the year 2000." They would, therefore, narrow the range of medical interest to more obvious pathology.

Leon Kass (1975) wonders at the loss of the physician's identity as he is mysteriously transmuted into a "member of the helping professions." Kass defines health in a narrow way, as a sort of physiologic and anatomic capacity for efficient functioning. To use medicine for any other goal than this, even when this goal is itself intrinsically valuable, is for Kass a "perversion of the art" of medicine.

Others have argued for strict limitations on a definition of health because of limitations on the availability of medical care. There is little enough medical care available, they claim, without "wasting" it on non-essentials such as elective abortions or sterilizations when contraception could be easily substituted.

The implicit assumption underlying both Kass's position and that of those arguing from considerations of scarce resources is that medicine must prevent or treat that which is unhealth and ignore that which is not. Those who propose a broader definition of health often seem to share this assumption. The battle by those who treat alcoholics to be labelled "mental health specialists" and to have alcoholism considered a disease may be an example of this. One of the primary motivations for this reclassification seems to be a desire to move into the aura of respectability that "Medicine" provides.

I think this model of doctors fighting disease and disease being that which doctors fight is overly simplistic. Kass is concerned that "since an endless profession is an ended profession, there will be an end to medicine unless there remains an end for" it. But surely a profession may pursue more than one goal. Lawyers seek due process under the law for their clients, but they also go into politics and legislate in accordance with higher standards. Musicians strive for aesthetic purity, but they may also try to please or educate their listeners. There does not seem to be any reason why medicine must be the only discipline to blind itself to its vast and multifaceted potential in mindless pursuit of a single goal. Why for instance, cannot doctors perform sterilizations even if such procedures do not promote health?

I think that once we disavow the alleged equivalence between conditions of unhealth and conditions which ought to be treated medically we will also find concepts of health and disease mush easier to mainipulate. Much of our confusion over what medicine is for and what health includes may vanish when we eliminate the moral overtones implicit in our use of these notions and acknowledge that medicine need not particularly be *for* anything. We need to reject the normative implications of diagnosis and to remodel the

doctor-patient relationship so that it is directed at the
needs of its participants rather than toward an arbitrary
external goal.

What I am arguing for, in a sense, is a sort of medical
freedom between consenting adults in the privacy of the
doctor's office of hospital ward. Clearly this medical
freedom will require constraints to keep it within socially
acceptable bounds, just as sexual liberty does. These will
mostly consist of assurances that the interests of other
concerned parties will be guarded. Family, friends, or
significant others may be entitled to some input into
decisions that effect them. Consider how much more difficult it would be to perform an abortion or sterilization
on a woman whose spouse was violently opposed to this, or
how much more problematic our case of rational suicide becomes because the man's Catholic wife objects and brings
him to the Emergency Room.

Society as a whole may also have legitimate concerns
impinging on the doctor-patient interaction. We will discuss some of these concerns in our topic on Cost Effectiveness and Patient Welfare.

Perhaps most importantly and most frequently overlooked,
the doctor himself may be entitled to some input into the
decision-making process, not as an MD but as a person, for
a doctor is someone with an MD who behaves in certain ways.
But a person with an MD has other roles to play than doctor.
He may be a friend, a taxpayer, a member of society. He
may also have relevant personal values, dedicated to patient
autonomy or a devout Catholic with profound religious
scruples about birth control and euthanasia. I think that,
at least except for emergencies, the physician generally
has a right to say, "These things I shall not do, even if
they might be proper for another."

How much input should be contributed to medical
decision-making by the patient, the physician, friends,
family or society I leave to you. This will probably vary
with circumstances. It may well be that rather than one
ideal model of medical decision-making there is a range of
acceptable practice. But medicine must be viewed not as a
crusade for health but as a tool, a body of knowledge or
skills which should be used for the benefit of those concerned. Like a gun, a printing press, or atomic power,

medicine is itself morally neutral. What we do or refuse to do with it is up to us and must not be blamed on an artificial "natural end of medicine."

What I have presented here this morning is my opinion. It is a carefully considered and hopefully rational opinion, and one which I believe I could defend on more fundamental grounds in another setting with more time, but it is an opinion nonetheless. Therefore, I do not urge it upon you. I only ask that you consider it, just as I ask that you consider some of the other concepts I have touched upon and still other thoughts that you will here today from speakers and fellow participants. To paraphrase an old cliche, none of us can provide you with *the* answers, but we can urge upon you lots of good questions. Think on them, and the answers you devise will help you with the individual dilemmas each of you may face tomorrow as well as with the cases you will discuss today.

REFERENCES

Kass, L (1975). Regarding the end of medicine and the
    pursuit of health. Public Interest 40 (summer): 11-41.
Redlich, FC (ed). (1976). "Concepts of health and disease".
    Special issue. J Med Phil 1 (3).
World Health Organization (1946). Constitution of the
    world health organization. Reprinted in Beauchamp TL,
    Childress JF (1979). "Principles of biomedical ethics."
    New York: Oxford University Press.

INTRODUCTION: THE REFUSAL TO STERILIZE

Marc D. Basson

Director, CEHM
University of Michigan
Ann Arbor, Michigan

The case in this topic is a simple one, quiet and
undramatic. No one is dying or being forced to live in
agony against his will. No ignorant or distraught patient
is being overruled or manipulated into an unsafe experiment.
The doctor does nothing irreversible to the patient and the
patient surely can find someone else to perform the tubal
ligation she seeks. Yet the discussion on this topic ranked
among the most heated that has ever occurred at one of the
conferences in this series. Several times it threatened to
degenerate into a shouting match.

Much of the controversy seemed to stem from the use of
"paternalistic" in the subtitle for this case. (The topic's
full title was "The Refusal to Sterilize: A Paternalistic
Decision".) Paternalism has become one of the buzz words of
bioethics, for despite the lack of agreement on the word's
precise meaning, to call something paternalistic is to
establish a prima facie moral case against it, based on
"patient rights", another recently emerged buzz word.

Tom Beauchamp attempts in his paper to describe what
consensus has emerged on the nature of paternalism. He
distinguishes between "strong paternalism", the overriding
of a rational, competent, and informed patient for his own
good, and "weak paternalism" in which the decision to override is justified by an attempt to disqualify the patient as
incompetent. This may be accomplished by casting aspersions
on the patient's intelligence, knowledge, or rationality.
Beauchamp points out that weak paternalism is clearly acceptable in at least some cases, but also doubts that this so-

called weak paternalism is indeed paternalistic in any interesting way. He is more interested in strong paternalism, which he takes to be an unjustified infringement of patient autonomy.

Eric Cassell has contributed an imaginative first person narrative which seems to attempt what Beauchamp views as a paternalistic justification for a refusal to sterilize. Cassell recounts details of "his" previous relationship with the Stanley family and tries to show how someone as rational and competent as Elizabeth Stanley seems might nonetheless really be motivated by highly charged emotions to the extent of refusing to engage in rational discourse.

Beauchamp would argue (and did, during the conference debate) that this is clearly paternalistic, that Cassell is refusing Elizabeth (whom Beauchamp says is as competent as anyone could be expected to be) for what he views as her own good. Cassell responds to such criticisms in this paper by denying the applicability of the notion of paternalism to the present case. He claims that it is too narrow to be relevant to the rich complexity of the doctor-patient relationship. Cassell also notes that since Elizabeth can always get her tubes tied elsewhere (not specified in the case), his refusal is only a decision for himself and not for Elizabeth. Thus, Cassell claims that his refusal cannot be construed as paternalistic.

For an approach to such problems very different from that of Cassell but still that of a clinical practitioner, the reader may wish to compare Cassell's paper with that of psychiatrist Jerome Motto on rational suicide elsewhere in this volume.

Rights and Responsibilities in Modern Medicine: The Second
Volume in a Series on Ethics, Humanism, and Medicine:135–136
© 1981 Alan R. Liss, Inc., 150 Fifth Avenue, New York, NY 10011

THE REFUSAL TO STERILIZE: A PATERNALISTIC DECISION

Case for Discussion

Elizabeth Stanley is a healthy, twenty-six-year-old
intern in Internal Medicine at Elsewhere County Medical
Center. Although she has been sexually active for several
years with different partners, she states that she has not
had the time or energy to socialize or meet men since coming
to Elsewhere County five months ago. She comes to the GYN
clinic today requesting a tubal ligation. She has never been
pregnant.

You are the staff gynecologist on service this month.
You have known Elizabeth and her family for years and were
influential in convincing her to come to Elsewhere County.
Somewhat taken aback, you ask her to elaborate on her reasons
for this request. She says that she is certain that she
never wants children and does not particularly care for any
of the available contraceptive techniques after exploring
then thoroughly.

Upon further questioning, she insists that she has
been thinking about this for several months and that she is
not considering that a tubal ligation might be reversible.
You suggest to her that if she ever marries, her husband
might want children. She replies, "then I won't marry him.
Or I can always adopt." She admits that there is a remote
chance that she might change her mind but says that she
thinks this unlikely. "Besides," she adds, "I want to make
sure I never reconsider. Having children would be unfair to
them and would get in the way of my career." She speaks
quietly but sincerely.

She would like to have her surgery in two weeks when she has been scheduled for a vacation. She says she came to the clinic this month because she has been very impressed with you and wants you to do her surgery.

What are your obligations as Elizabeth's friend? As her physician? What is the purpose of modern medicine and is the requested procedure consistent with it? Do you feel disturbed by Elizabeth's attempt to bind a future self to childlessness irreversibly?

**Rights and Responsibilities in Modern Medicine: The Second
Volume in a Series on Ethics, Humanism and Medicine: 137—143**
© 1981 Alan R. Liss, Inc., 150 Fifth Avenue, New York, NY 10011

PATERNALISM AND REFUSALS TO STERILIZE

Tom L. Beauchamp

Georgetown University

Washington, D.C.

I shall begin by discussing the issue of paternalism,
returning later to the case before us. Under the "issue of
paternalism," as it is reflected in the philosophical literature on the subject, I include antipaternalism (or the position
defended by those opposed to all forms of paternalism) as well
as certain important distinctions such as that between strong
and weak paternalism. The latter distinction is of critical
importance for our purposes in analyzing the case of Elizabeth
Stanley.

There are reasons for thinking that paternalism is a pervasive feature of modern society. Governmental agencies such
as the Food and Drug Administration are regarded by many, including some of its own members, as inherently paternalistic.
The profession of medicine too is often hailed as a paternalistic institution, especially in the relationship between
patients and physicians. Illness, injury, depression, fear,
threat of death, and heavy dosages of drugs may overwhelm
patients, making them incompetent to know their best interests or to make reasonable judgments. At the very least they
are compromised in making judgments. Moreover, every increase
in illness or medication can increase patient dependence on
his or her physician. The medical profession thus seems to
many unable to escape a paternalistic orientation.

On the other hand, the paternalism of the medical profession has been under attack in recent years, especially by
defenders of patient choice and autonomy. They hold that
physicians intervene too often, treat moral and prudential
judgments as if they were medical judgments, and in general

assume too much control over patients' choices. Philosophers and lawyers persuaded of this view have tended to see the patient/physician relationship as grounded on patient autonomy, and a recent draft of principles of ethics by the American Medical Association asserts that "Paternalism in the profession is no longer appropriate." What is meant by this statement, and indeed what is meant in general by "paternalism," is confusing. Why the case of Elizabeth Stanley should be construed as paternalistic is no less confusing, as we shall see. For these reasons, I will pursue the topic of the nature of paternalism a bit further.

The word "paternalism" is loosely used to refer to practices of treating individuals in the way a father treats his children. When this analogy is applied to medical professionals, two features of the paternal role are involved: 1) the father's beneficence (the presumption that the interests of his children are paramount) and 2) the father's role in making decisions (he makes decisions pertaining to his children's welfare, rather than letting them make the decisions). Paternalism poses moral questions because beneficence toward others can take precedence over the autonomous wishes or actions of those persons. For example, in the case that we have before us, should the doctor choose to override the autonomous choice of Elizabeth Stanley? If so, should this be done because it is in her best interest that this course be taken (rather than a way of protecting the moral integrity of the consulting physician)? A paternalistic decision to override autonomous choice results from any affirmative answer. The major question we have before us (at least if we accept the way paternalistic issues are generally framed) is "When are paternalistic reasons ever good enough reasons for the limitation of individual liberty?" If one accepts a paternalistic principle then limitation of personal liberty can be justified if through acts of personal liberty one would produce serious harm to oneself. I want to emphasize that the restrictions must actually be liberty limiting where liberty is expressed through rational choices; otherwise (conceptually or by definition) a restriction cannot be paternalistic.

The moral problem, then, is that of whether it is ethically justified for one party to override the liberty of action or choices of another party when the reason for the restriction of liberty is purely paternalistic. Many actions, rules, and laws are commonly justified by appeal to some form of the paternalistic principle. Examples in medicine include court orders for blood transfusions when patients refuse them, involuntary commitment to institutions for treatment, intervention to stop "rational" suicides, and resuscitating patients who have asked not to be resuscitated. Hospital policies and even procedures adopted by individual physicians can be paternalistic in this sense.

A paternalism of the description just provided has been defended in an influential article by Gerald Dworkin, who argues that paternalism should be regarded as a form of social insurance policy that fully rational individuals would take out in order to protect themselves. Such persons would know, for example, that they might be tempted at times to make decisions that are potentially dangerous and irreversible, and they might at other times be pressured to do something they deep down believe too risky--such as reacting to the social pressures involved in being challenged to a fight by someone. Dworkin's views might be applied to the case before us, for certain kinds of pressures play a role in leading Elizabeth Stanley toward what her physician regards as a premature conclusion. In related cases, Dworkin believes that persons might not understand and appreciate the facts about research on smoking, even after hearing extensive public health education information on the subject. Again, one might argue that Elizabeth Stanley is unable to appreciate the radical nature of her decision at her present level of maturity. Instead of informing persons of facts or teaching them to appreciate the facts, which may not always be possible, Dworkin concludes that all rational persons would agree to a limited grant of power to others to control their actions.

For the aforementioned reasons, the case of Elizabeth Stanley seems a candidate for justified paternalism of the sort recommended by Dworkin. Her decision would be irreversible; she is apparently under significant career pressures; and she may well be quite immature (and partially ignorant of her future desires), despite her education and profession.

Having introduced paternalism and its justification, I now turn to antipaternalism and the reasons why some have held that the principle of paternalism is not a valid principle for restricting liberty under any circumstances. Two main reasons have been offered in support of this position. The first reason is that a broad range of adverse consequences will accrue by giving paternalistic powers to the state and to medical officials. In other words, if you grant them a valid paternalistic principle then pervasive abuse will follow from the use of that principle. Paternalistic principles are said to be too broad, and hence, to justify too much restriction of liberty. This reason is used by antipaternalists together with a second reason-- namely, the significance of violations of autonomy inherently involved in paternalistic interferences. The antipaternalist typically holds that the autonomous individual is almost always in a position to ascertain his or her own best interests more competently than anyone else, including instances where the professional opinions of physicians are involved.

I want now to move to the distinction I mentioned previously between strong and weak paternalism, an extremely important distinction for discussions of medical paternalism. Weak paternalism holds that an individual engaging in self-regarding conduct can be restricted only when it is a substantially nonvoluntary act; thus you can only justifiably interfere with someone's "liberty" if they are in a substantially nonvoluntary state. Persons under the influence of psychotropic drugs, or in a condition of painful labor while delivering a child, or suffering from a blow on the head affecting memory and judgment are examples of persons in medical situations who have their voluntary capacities limited. Presumably cases where consent is given but the consenting party is inadequately informed are also instances of actions where voluntariness is critically impaired. Effectively, then, weak paternalism is the view that a person's autonomy or liberty may be limited because his or her capacity for autonomous action is severely limited and someone else knows their interests better than they do themselves, at least in their current condition.

Strong paternalism, by contrast, holds that it is sometimes justified to protect or benefit a person by limiting choices or actions even when the person's contrary choices or actions are substantially voluntary and informed. The strong paternalist says that even in circumstances where persons are not particularly compromised by their conditions you can still validly override their self-regarding choices and actions. The grounds are that some agents capable of autonomous decisions do not know their own best interests despite possessing adequate information about their situation and despite being substantially voluntary. Strong paternalists would often intervene, for example, to stop an autonomous person from committing suicide and would require everyone to wear seatbelts for their health and safety.

Major problems about paternalism are generated by this distinction between strong and weak paternalism. Virtually everyone acknowledges that some acts normally conceived as weak paternalistic acts are justified, including even many antipaternalists. For example: Let us suppose that a person is enjoying the influence of LSD and takes it in mind to commit suicide. Under such an influence, so far as I can see, nobody believes that it is unjustified to intervene. One might infer, as weak paternalists do, that if some forms of paternalism are clearly justified, then antipaternalism is just as clearly mistaken. Here the problem with paternalism for ethical theory is reduced to that of deciding which form of (justified) paternalism is correct. In other words, if you can find one example of a justified paternalism, then antipaternalism is clearly false. The only remaining problem would be to discover which form of paternalism is correct--at least this is the way much of the most influential literature on paternalism has developed the issue.

The difficulty with this position, however, is that weak paternalism may not be paternalism in any interesting sense, for the "actions" involved seem beyond the knowledge and control of the "actors"--that is, the actions seem substantially nonvoluntary and substantially uninformed due to conditions beyond the knowledge and control of the "actors." Who, after all, would leave unprotected from medical intervention defenseless children, those who are mentally retarded, those suffering from severe pain, and those who have so little information about their case that they completely misunderstand their situation? The answer, of course, is that no caring or sane person would defend this point of view, and thus the paternalist has a fairly easy time of painting antipaternalists as radicals who mistake their successful rejection of strong paternalism for a successful wholesale rejection of all forms of paternalism, and so as a successful refutation of weak paternalism.

If this argument were correct, then antipaternalists would be defending both a detestable and a confused position, for they would have simply confused strong paternalism and weak paternalism. But is this paternalistic argument correct? In my judgment, it is seriously confused and incorrect. The antipaternalist is not defending the position that the actions

of intervening which the weak paternalism <u>believes to be
justified</u> are in fact <u>unjustified</u>. That is a mistaken
characterization of antipaternalism. On the contrary, the
antipaternalist agrees that these interventions are justified,
but the antipaternalist sees them as justifiied <u>because</u> the
so-called actions or choices of the agent are substantially
nonvoluntary in all important respects. The paternalist
thus seems to me to have misconceived the issue. The weak
paternalist and the antipaternalist should agree, for they
defend exactly the same position. Thus, I think the only
interesting position is the position of the strong paternalist, namely that the liberty of persons can be validly over-
ridden when they are substantially autonomous and substantially informed.

Let me now try to apply all this to the case of Elizabeth
Stanley. Elizabeth Stanley is described as a healthy 26-year
old intern, apparently competent and capable of autonomous decisions. As far as I can see, she is as capable of autonomous
decisions as the so-called "reasonable person" in the law.
Her reasons are that she never wants children and does not
care for the contraceptive alternatives, after exploring them
thoroughly. You may think her reasons weak and foolish and
without adequate foresight, yet she has been thinking about
her situation for some time, is far from simply walking in
off the street, and she knows that when her tubes are tied
the procedure would not be reversible. She speaks quietly in
the course of the interview, sincerely, and with conviction
about her case. Any intervention to prevent her from carrying
out her wishes under the circumstance seems to me would have
to be <u>strong</u> paternalism, not weak paternalism, and I take it
that the weak paternalist and the antipaternalist would con-
cur. They would both say in this case that an intervention
is not justified. This means that in order to justify an intervention strong paternalism must be accepted. Since I know
of no defense of strong paternalism that is adequate, I regard the intervention as unjustified.

I can think of only one somewhat engaging line that might
be taken by the paternalist in this circumstance. The position
is the following: Elizabeth Stanley is asking another physician
to compromise his or her moral principles by performing a procedure which he or she strongly believes ill-advised. Since
no one ought to be required to act against their morally considered conscientious beliefs, at most such a physician has a
moral obligation to <u>refer</u> Elizabeth to another physician from

whom she can receive further assistance. This position, however, faces a considerable dilemma. The dilemma is the following: If the physician is merely making an appeal to conscience, or to his or her moral integrity and right not to do
something considered morally repugnant, then this decision is
not paternalistic, and our whole motivation for examining
this case has vanished. However, if the physician's sole or
even major reason for resisting Elizabeth Stanley's request
is that his or her moral integrity or conscience would be
violated because Elizabeth Stanley stands to be harmed in the
future by her decision, then the position being defended is
paternalism, and indeed strong paternalism; for the physician
limits her liberty out of a belief that she will be harmed as
a result of her own freely chosen course. There could scarce-
ly be a more purely paternalistic motivation.

Rights and Responsibilities in Modern Medicine: The Second
Volume in a Series on Ethics, Humanism, and Medicine: 145–152
© 1981 Alan R. Liss, Inc., 150 Fifth Avenue, New York, NY 10011

THE REFUSAL TO STERILIZE ELIZABETH STANLEY IS NOT PATERNALISM

Eric J. Cassell, M.D.,F.A.C.P.
Cornell University Medical College
1300 York Avenue, New York, N.Y. 10021

Let me start with Elizabeth Stanley. I do
not believe that this is a case of paternalism.
Dr. Stanley would like a tubal ligation. I would
not like to ligate Elizabeth Stanley's fallopian
tubes. I am not the only surgeon in town and Liz
can go to another surgeon. I have not made a
decision for her, I have made a decision for me.

I knew Elizabeth's father from way back and
we were in the Army together in an infantry unit
around Salerno that had a bad time for a few
days. He died when Liz was still in high school
but we had always kept in touch. He was a good
man whom I owe a favor, dead or not. So when she
came here before her internship and spoke to me I
thought that she was Arnold's kid and part of my
skin. When I looked at her I could see Arnold. I
couldn't really but I was so glad knowing that
she was a doctor and would be at County. I was
really happy about it. So when she came in the
first time to talk about the tubal I was totally
unprepared. I wanted to tell her about her father
and about what we all wanted, and hoped for, and
talked about endlessly because we were even
younger than she is. You know, the way you would
talk to the child of a friend who was old enough
to know something and to joke and talk about wars
and parents and training programs. Someone who
was at the same time your child and not your
child. A surgeon and a friend, but a young
friend. Anyway that was definitely not Elizabeth
Stanley. I got the whole tubal ligation number by
the Woman's Movement book. Every objection that I
offerred was countered not by any content but

merely by her telling me about her rights as an
individual--and also how I had let her down.
(Never entered her mind for even a moment that
she might have let me down ((to say nothing of
Arnold)). So after hearing her out (and feeling
like someone going back to the restaurant where
they ate the first great meal of their lives and
seeing cardboard arrive on the plate) I said that
I was sorry, but I was not going to tie her tubes
and that was the end of it. She said it was
certainly not the end of it. She had rights and
no paternalistic SOB was going to ruin her life
whether he knew her father or not. That was what
Ethics Committees were for and we would discuss
it next in front of the commmittee. To tell you
the honest truth, all the substantive matters
about having children or not, reversibility or
not, surgical risk or not, the actual factual
basis for her desire to become infertile got lost
in the yelling that followed my saying NO. So we
don't misunderstand each other, I am not about to
sterilize Arnold's kid just because as a green
no-nothing intern who has had loose bowels,
sweaty hands and no sleep for a month, she thinks
that is the way she is going to show the world
that she is grown-up. Okay, I may not know why
she wants to do it but I don't think she does
either. There isn't a doctor in the world who
does not know that people change their minds.
When decisions are made that have permanent
effects and could be put off, I think it is
perfectly reasonable to require that enough time
pass to insure that the person has given the
decision sufficient thought. That is not the case
here. So I think if she wants to get her tubes
tied let her wait a year. If she gets pregnant
before then I will happily abort her. Meanwhile,
why do I have to act as if every thought that
crossed the mind of every person--female or not,
doctor or not, had the same weight as the Magna
Carta. Let them do what they want and me do what
I want. As long as mine is not the final
determinant than it is simply not paternalism.

Elizabeth's biggest gripe with me seemed to
be that I did not respect her rights as an

individual. I thought that If I heard the word
'individual' once more I was going to hemorrhage.
She kept telling me about her rights as an
individual and I kept asking her what she meant
by the word 'individual'. Not surprisingly she
never did define it. It is an interesting thing
about medical schools and training programs that
they teach an enormous amount about disease,
pathophysiology, and all the sciences from
anatomy to xerography that back up our knowledge
about disease but nowhere do they teach what a
patient is. I suppose the reason is that it is
considered self-evident what a patient is.

Like so many other self-evident concepts,
this one also deserves some thought. A patient
is, of course, a person. That is another
seemingly obvious word whose meaning is somewhat
obscure. You will not find the term in a medical
dictionary! My daughter once said "I am not a
servant and I am not a child--I am a PERSON!"
(her declaration, not surprisingly, was in the
context of washing the dishes). I said "You are
telling me what a person is not, Justine, but
what IS a person." She like the rest of us was
not too clear on the matter. Failing a definition
of person, we fall back on the word 'individual'.

Since I am not a philosopher, I am not
qualified to talk about the concept of individual
except as it expresses itself in the way most
people talk and act in regard to it. In the
American heritage the concept of the individual
seems extraordinarily important. (Actually the
word 'person' is used in the Constitution
interchangably with the word 'individual'.) But
as far as I can tell the derivation of the term,
even as it is most often used in medicine, is
primarily political. In which case we speak of
the individual VERSUS the state, or VERSUS
another individual. In those contexts what is
usually being referred to are the rights of
individuals, or their obligations, and so on.
That is the way Elizabeth Stanley used the term
when she spoke about her right to have a tubal
ligation. Stanley Hauerwas told me that the word

'individual' was originally a term in logic
referring to unity which was then borrowed by the
political philosophers of the Enlightenment.

It seems to me that to be an individual in
the sense that it is most often used in this
country is only one aspect of being a person--but
by no means the only aspect. Further, as I noted
earlier, in the sense it is usually used it is a
political concept. Clearly all persons have a
political facet--that is they are members of a
state, a government, a civil unit, or some other
polity, but most of us would not like to be
defined SOLELY by our political aspect. Elizabeth
Stanley was quite definite about it being a
political matter. She was sure that my refusal to
sterilize her was not only paternalistic, but a
repressive stance against women as a group. In
that sense what seemed to me to be a personal
matter was to her political because of its
implications for the group.

Hidden within the word 'individual' are two
conflicting meanings. And further, that conflict,
hidden as it may be, has sharpened in recent
decades. The political meaning of the word
individual is indifferent to individual
differences. An individual has rights regardless
of gender, color, ethnic group, religion and
also regardless of whether he or she is tall or
short, fat or thin, fast or slow or even with or
without glucose-6-phosphate dehydrogenase. That
is odd because if a physician was indifferent to
individual differences while treating sick
people, disaster would follow. That is because
things like stature, weight, gender, even
religion and ethnic group have an effect on the
presentation, clinical course, treatment and
outcome of illness. I know very well that when
Dr. Stanley was speaking about her rights as an
individual she meant that aspect of herself that
has no individuality. Merely herself as a free
standing entity was what (or who) was
entitled to the tubal ligation. But there is
something basically paradoxical about that demand
because a tubal ligation has very personal

meanings. (I will return to the word 'personal' shortly.)

The two conflicting meanings of the word individual, one indifferent to individual differences and the other solely concerned with differences, cause greater trouble now, I believe, than at any time in the history of the word. Because this is an era of Radical Individuality, or another term might be Radical Autonomy. A time where individual in the sense of individual differences has achieved its greatest importance. I matter nowadays not only because I am an individual versus the government or another individual or group, but because I am ME! With all the talents, skills, failings, hopes, desires, aspirations, anxieties, concerns, needs, and etc. etc. that make up the unique individual that is me. But now we have come upon another paradox. ME, with all those desires, fears, hopes, etc. cannot be seen apart from my past, my parents, my training, my friends, my country, my traditions because the ME that I AM is inseparable from those other things.

When I the individual becomes ME, I leave the almost statistical configuration of the political individual and become a person. A person is a very complex complex. A person contains within himself or herself: A lived past, a family's lived past, culture and society, roles, the political individual, associations, an unconscious, a body and relationships to it, day to day behaviors, a private inner life, a hoped for future, and perhaps more.

So when I was talking to Elizabeth Stanley about a tubal ligation-- when any physician considers an ethical issue in medicine, he or she cannot be content with individual (in the political sense) or Radical Autonomy, what must always be harkened back to are those flesh and blood real persons that are our concern of whom only one part is the individual in a political sense. (I think it is fair to say that our whole nation is having trouble squaring the two different meanings of the word individual. We are justly proud of our heritage of individual liberties but we simply do not know how to deal with the fact that some individuals are better or worse at some things than others and to treat everybody as though they have the same talents because they have the same rights does a great disservice to those with lesser abilities.)

If that is what a person is, then what is a patient? A patient is a sick person. As sick modifies person linguistically, so sickness modifies a person in real life. It is a fundamental error to consider a sick person the same as a well person but with a disease stuck on the side--much as the person would carry a knapsack. Illness, as anybody knows who works with the sick or who has ever really been sick, can change behavior, thinking, or judgement (as well as a lot of other things). As Milton Erikson said " It is a matter of common knowledge often overlooked, disregarded or rejected that a patient can be silly, forgetful, absurd, unreasonable, illogical, incapable of acting with commen sense, and very often governed and directed in his behavior by emotions and by unknowm, unrecognizable, and perhaps undiscoverable unconscious needs and forces which are far from reasonable. logical or sensible."

The solution to the ethical problems in medicine raised by those potential characteristics of patienthood is not to pretend that they are untrue. That might be good philosophy, but it is bad medicine. The difficulty is increased by the fact that when patients start to become all those things that Erikson describes, no light goes on over their head to announce the fact. They may look and sound just as reasonable as they did instants previously. What should we do about those characteristics of the sick person? The medical response of times past was to assume control over the decision making as though the patient was oncapable. That is what is called paternalism and it is justly condemned. An alternative response

by physicians is the abdication of
responsibility. That is what physicians do who
pretend that a sick person is the same in
everyway as a well person. Of course the sick
person is still an individual in the political
sense of having rights (and obligations) but not
necessarily in the ability to exercise those
rights. A better response than either paternalism
or the abdication of responsibilty is an new
understanding of the function of medicine. Here
the job of the physician is to help the patient
maintain his or her autonomy to the degree
possible in the face of illness. Gerald Dworkin
defined autonomy as being made up of authenticity
and independance. It is clear that physicians
have the ability to help the patient maintain his
or her authenticity in the face of illness.
Equally they have the capacity to destroy
authenticity. In the same manner they can
enhance or destroy the patient's
independance--freedom of choice, by how they
provide information for decision making or
facilitate the patient's ability to act in his or
her own best interests. Physicians' capacities in
these regards imply not only their acceptance of
those responsibilities, but something special
about their relationship with their patients.
Indeed, the doctor-patient relationship does
carry within it the potential for the physician
to act as true agent for the patient in the
battle against sickness.

Space does not permit me to go into detail,
but several things about the relationship must be
made clear. It is possible for the physician to
blend his or her knowledge of the body and
disease with the knowledge acquired about the
patient so that decisions can be made by the
patient that are authentic to the patient--not
merely what the physician thinks the patient
wants. Learning how to do that requires training
and experience, but most of all it requires
acknowledging the importance of such shared
decisions. Further, the relationship between
doctor and patient occurs over time and involves
changes in the patient's capacities, the doctor's

knowledge and the relationship itself. The doctor-patient relationship is little understood in part because the society has laid such stress on the individual that there has not been a consonant growth in our knowledge of such relations. But lack of understanding should not diminish our respect for its power or importance in the care of the sick.

In the light of all that do you wonder that I refused Elizabeth's request to tie her tubes. I may never accede simply because I think she is wrong and in the final analysis it is my act, not merely her decision, that must be judged. But her framework of analysis, based as it is on individual rights--the individual as a political entity, is entirely inadequate to her decision. The individual in that sense of the term is but one part of a person and the tubal ligation involves the entire person. So does the care of the sick.

DISCUSSION SUMMARY: THE REFUSAL TO STERILIZE

Marc D. Basson

Director, CEHM
University of Michigan
Ann Arbor, Michigan

Many of the participants questioned Elizabeth Stanley's
motivation and certainty, noting the irreversibility of the
decision and her insistence on having the procedure done soon.
They also commented on the likely impairment of her decision-
making ability by the stress of internship. Assuming that
they had satisfied themselves as to these points, the participants were almost unanimous that the doctor had to either
refer Elizabeth to another competent gynecologist who might
operate or to perform the tubal ligation himself. They felt
that Elizabeth's apparent intelligence and fund of knowledge
certainly qualified her to give an informed consent and that
the proper role of the physician was to help Elizabeth direct
her own life.

The discussants were less certain whether the unwilling
gynecologist was himself obligated to do the sterilization.
About 80 percent of the participants felt that the doctor
ought to refuse because of his own belief that the ligation
was not indicated. "If a doctor is morally opposed to a
practice," commented one, "then he ought to act on his convictions." Most did not see a contradiction in saying that
the doctor should refer the patient to someone else but
should not do it himself. "This much is owed to the patient
out of respect for his values," commented one lawyer.
About 15 percent said they would do the surgery even though
they thought the idea foolish. "She is a mature and independent woman and has the right to make her own decisions,
even stupid ones," a physician stated. "I offer my services
and advice to patients, but I would no more force the latter
on a patient than the former." Finally, five percent of the

participants simply refused to indicate a decision despite pressure to do so.

INTRODUCTION: COST EFFECTIVENESS AND PATIENT WELFARE

Marc D. Basson

Director, CEHM
University of Michigan
Ann Arbor, Michigan

There was a time when the only public policy problem related to the distribution of health care was how to build enough hospitals and train enough staff to go around. It was the era of the doctor shortage, when every American had a right to health care and it was society's obligation to satisfy all medical needs.

Today all has changed. Economists now tell us that the demand for health care may be inexhaustible while our pocketbooks and the Gross National Product are not. Rather than finding money to buy new equipment for our hospitals, we now strive to force them to make do with what they have. Without a Certificate of Need, administrators are not permitted to spend money on new scanners or hospital wings. Once, the government grandly proclaimed that it would pay for any patient who needed dialysis. This year, government officials decided to discontinue reimbursements for heart transplants. The trustees of Massachusetts General Hospital have voted not to allow their Department of Surgery to do heart transplants, not because they are unreliable but because they are not cost effective.

Meredith Eiker and Norman Daniels both approach the problems of spiralling health care costs and increasingly unrealistic popular expectations from this new point of view. Both seem to agree that the growth of the health care industry must be limited. They differ on how this goal ought to be achieved, however.

Norman Daniels is a philosopher who has long been interested in questions of social justice and distribution of resources. His premise is that all deserve equal initial access to health care and that this must be achieved by some sort of macro-allocative redistribution scheme. His plan would then leave the individual doctor and patient free to pursue the best health care that can be achieved within this framework. (Daniels assumes, in order to simplify his analysis, that physicians and patients all share the same views as to what constitutes optimal care. A fuller analysis would have to take this into account.)

In the course of her training in public health and hospital administration, Meredith Eiker has come to believe that the true culprit for rising health care costs is the public that keeps increasing its demands and expectations. She attacks the view that the health care industry itself should be responsible for cost-cutting as irresponsible, for supply increases in proportion to demand. For the same reason, she believes it important that we not cut costs on the macro level by reducing supply and yet encourage the demands of individual patients and physicians on the micro level to remain unchecked. She proposes that we force consumers of health care to make their own individual scarce resource allocation decisions by rationing out to each a fixed and equal amount of available health care, per year or for life. In this way, Eiker argues, the patient himself will be motivated to curtail his demands in order to "save up" health care for possible future needs. Eiker prefaces her suggestion with the statement that it seems permissible to ration other scarce national resources and therefore skips over the chief argument that may be raised against any rationing. This is that individual liberties to purchase the good in question may be more important than the national good to be achieved.

Eiker's plan is obviously oversimplified, containing, for instance, no provision for catastrophic illness, but it is meant more as a challenge than a serious proposal as it is stated here. After all, why not do this, she seems to ask. And for those who think it might be appropriate, there is the greatest public policy challenge of all: deciding how.

Rights and Responsibilities in Modern Medicine: The Second
Volume in a Series on Ethics, Humanism, and Medicine: 157—158
© 1981 Alan R. Liss, Inc., 150 Fifth Avenue, New York, NY 10011

COST EFFECTIVENESS AND PATIENT WELFARE

Case for Discussion

The guaiac test is an inexpensive qualitative test for
minute amounts of blood. A positive stool guaiac may be
caused by many things, including hemorrhoids and benign
intestinal polyps. However, one major cause of positive
stool guaiacs is colonic cancer. This is a curable disease
if diagnosed sufficiently early. Thus, most hospital-based
physicians routinely perform this test on patients as they
are admitted. A positive stool guaiac in the absence of
obvious cause is generally considered a cause for further
investigation designed to rule out cancer.

In 1974, the American Cancer Society endorsed a protocol
involving six sequential stool guaiacs as a screen for
colorectal cancer. Since any single stool guaiac detects
only about 92% of such cancers, presumably more would be
picked up by two than by one, more by three than two, and so
forth.

Unfortunately the cost also increases. In 1975,
Neuhauser and Lewicki worked out an elaborate cost-benefit
analysis for stool guaiac screening. They assumed that doing
a stool guaiac test costs $4.00, including the test material
and "indirect costs arising from teaching and implementing
the diet and testing procedure." They assumed that each
additional test would only cost $1.00 since the patient had
already been instructed and placed on his diet. They then
compared the results of the one test screen with the multiple
test screens. They found that when multiple tests were performed fewer cases of cancer were found with a second guaiac
than with the first, fewer still with a third test, and so

forth.   Thus, while multiple test screens do lead to the
diagnosis of slightly more cancer patients, the marginal cost per patient diagnosed mounts rapidly with the number
of tests performed; for one test screening, $1,175 per case
diagnosed ; for two test screening, $5,492; for a three test
screen, $49,724,965.   For a full six test screening program,
the cost per additional diagnosed case would be $47,107,214.

The point of this case is to study ethics, not statistics.
Therefore assume the validity of the figures above.   How many
guaiacs would you ask your staff physicians to perform?   If
you were a patient, how many would you want performed on you?
If these answers are different, how would you resolve the conflict between them?   How many stool guaiacs ought a physician
to perform?   How much is a human life worth?

**Rights and Responsibilities in Modern Medicine: The Second
Volume in a Series on Ethics, Humanism, and Medicine: 159–170**
© 1981 Alan R. Liss, Inc., 150 Fifth Avenue, New York, NY 10011

COST-EFFECTIVENESS AND PATIENT WELFARE[1]

Norman Daniels

Tufts University

Medford, Massachusetts

Does the employment of cost-effectiveness or cost-
benefit methodologies in determining which medical treatment
is delivered violate the rights or entitlements of patients?
Even if no rights or entitlements are infringed, is it
morally wrong to employ these methodologies as part of our
resource allocation methodology? I will try to sketch an
answer to these rather general questions before turning to
some specific problems with these methodologies themselves
and to the issues raised by the Neuhauser & Lewicki studies,
(1973, 1976) which provide the basis for our case study.

I shall begin by sketching what I think is a fairly
widely held--though not uncontroversial--view of the role of
the physician. On this view the physician is seen as having
entered into a relationship with a specific patient which
binds him to acting in the best interests of the patient,
with the patient's consent, of course. One important product
the physician delivers to the patient is reassurance and
what is somewhat romantically called "caring." No doubt this
is an important part of the notion of 'quality' of care. But
I here want to leave it out of the picture, at the risk of
oversimplifying my discussion. Instead, I want to focus on
another feature of the product the physician delivers, namely
a package of services--diagnostic and therapeutic--which
carry with them various benefits, harms, and risks. Suppose
we consider a simplified conception of this package and
assume it can be expressed as a sum of benefits and burdens

[1]Research for this paper was supported by Grant No.HS03097
from the National Center for Health Services Research, OASH.

(including risks). And let us for the moment not consider
monetary costs among the burdens to anyone--patients or
society. We are focusing on the medical impact of the
"benefits minus burdens" package. We might try to express
this whole package in monetary terms--which of course
raises questions about just how to do so. But let me for
the moment leave this conversion aside. The notion I have
characterized here corresponds, I believe, to what Avedis
Donabedian (1979, p.279-82) has called "absolute" quality.

The 'benefits minus burdens' package clearly varies
with the total quantity, as well as the selection, of
services. Since adding services does not always increase
the sum of benefits and burdens--we run into unnecessary,
iatrogenic services--we can imagine that 'absolute' quality
may have a maximum point when benefits-minus-burdens is
plotted against quantity of services, i.e., total monetary
costs of services. Clearly, absolute quality is a function
of the state of medical science, but, as Donabedian points
out, it also critically reflects "how well the science and
technology are used" (1979, p.280). Moreover, for any
ceiling on the volume of services, stated, say, in monetary
terms, the absolute quality of care will be maximal when the
sum of benefits-minus-burdens is greatest.

Using this idealized notion of absolute quality, we can
now restate the task of the physician according to the
traditional view. He is to act in the patient's best
interests, by making the patient aware of what treatment
package maximizes absolute quality, and if the patient agrees
to such treatment, to pursue it. Of course, from the
patient's perspective, the benefits-minus-burdens calculation
may come out differently. This is clearly the case if the
patient includes in the calculation his cost-sharing of the
monetary cost of the treatment package; but we might also
find patients evaluate the costs of lost time, pain, fear,
and so on according to their own utility functions or
preferences. In any case, the patient may be seen as trying
to maximize what Donabedian calls "individual quality," which
includes monetary costs to the patient. The task of the
physician then is to facilitate the patient in pursuing this
goal, informing him as fully as possible of the relevant
facts about absolute quality so the patient can make his own
adjustments. (This view of the patient as decision-maker is
clearly less tenable for very ill patients who want no such
burden). Let us assume, for the sake of simplicity, that

absolute and individual quality will differ primarily because of patient cost-sharing. So if patient cost-sharing is eliminated, as it is on some insurance schemes, we can imagine a coincidence of physician and patient goals with regard to the quality of care.

Now we can restate our main problem. Absolute quality will vary with the overall quantity of services available. If resource constraints keep the level of available services below the level that leads to an overall maximal absolute quality, then physicians and patients will have to settle for next-best solutions. One way to put our initial question would be to ask if limiting the search for absolute (or individual) quality to next best solutions is morally permissible, and if it is, what would justify such limitations? Or, is the patient _entitled_ to have the physician act on his behalf to utilize all resources necessary to maximizing absolute quality of care (assuming the patient's consent)?

I would like to factor out of this discussion, at least for the moment, the question of who pays for the treatment, for I think the central issue arises regardless of how the financing burden is distributed. Suppose, for example, all costs are borne by patients out of pocket. Then the question is whether the wealthiest patients, whom we may suppose can afford all treatments, should be entitled to purchase them, regardless of what the effects on resource allocation are elsewhere in the system? I think the answer is that if the demand induced by such entitlements would yield socially unacceptable resource problems elsewhere in the society, then there should be no such entitlements. (Of course, a system that avoids rationing in one way (budget ceilings) imposes it in another (ability to pay), a point I shall return to later.) So let us leave aside for the moment the question of who pays, remembering in any case that there is no free lunch. The question, again, is whether society is obliged to permit health care resources to be allocated purely in response to physician-patient intentions to maximize absolute care?

The obvious worry here is that resources are limited and that considerations of justice and efficiency may lead us to question the correctness of allocations made in response to the unrestrained pursuit of absolute quality. I will begin my attempt to answer by arguing first that there are some important social obligations, deriving from considerations of justice, to provide an adequate level of health care services and to make sure the services are equitably distributed. Here I can only sketch the core of a theory I elaborate elsewhere. [1] Suppose we ask what is specially important about health care compared to other social goods. Many people--in many societies--feel it _is_ specially important, for they often insist it be more equally (or equitably) distributed than various other social goods. What might explain its special importance?

We need to back up a bit and consider the function of health care. Suppose we adopt a rather narrow (if not uncontroversial) view of disease: diseases will be departures from normal species functioning. Health care needs, broadly construed, are things we need to prevent, maintain, restore, or compensate for departures from normal species functioning. Why are such departures from normal functioning of social importance? One initially plausible answer is that we need normal functioning whatever else we need or want--it is a necessary condition for happiness, say. But this answer seems less plausible when we note that happiness or satisfaction in life does not so clearly require normal functioning. Many people 'cope' well with significant impairments.

A more plausible answer, I believe, is that normal species functioning is an important determinant of the opportunity range open to individuals in a society. The opportunity range is the array of life plans reasonable to pursue within given conditions obtaining in a society. This range is, of course, relative to various social facts about the society--its stage of technological development, material well being, and so on. Thus, similar impairments of normal species functioning might have different effects on opportunity range in different societies. But within a society, it becomes possible to give at least a crude ranking to the effects of different impairments of normal func-

[1] I draw here on my "Health Care Needs and Distributive Justice," Philosophy and Public Affairs (forthcoming); this is part of a booklength project, Justice and Health Care Delivery, which will be published by Cambridge University Press.

tioning in terms of their effects on the normal opportunity range. In turn, this gives us a crude ranking of the importance of different health care needs.

I am suggesting that we can account for the special importance ascribed to health care needs by noting the connection between meeting those needs and the opportunity range open to individuals in a given society. This suggests that the principles of justice governing the distribution of health care should derive from our general principles of justice guaranteeing fair equality of opportunity (cf. Rawls, 1971, Sect.14). Specifically, health care institutions will be among a variety of basic institutions (e.g. educational ones) which are important because they insure that conditions of fair equality of opportunity obtain. I cannot here argue the issues in the general theory of justice that would support the view that fair equality of opportunity is a requirement of justice. But if I am granted the assumption that it is, we have the foundations for important social obligations in the distribution of health care.

There are, to be sure, worries about my approach. For example, the notion of opportunity has to be age-relativized or it seems to embody a significant age bias, like productivity measures of the value of life-saving technologies. Similarly, I must show that these requirements of justice do not open a bottomless pit into which we are required to pour endless resources in quest of an unreachable egalitarian goal. But this is not the place to consider even such important details, and I do discuss them elsewhere.

Instead it is more important to show some of the implications of this view for the distribution of health care. First, I think the theory implies a fairly strong principle of equal initial access to the health care system. If there is a social obligation to provide for equality of opportunity through the provision of important health care needs, then people must be in a position to have their needs assessed. This assessment requires access independent of geographical and financial barriers. Just what system of health care financing--what formula of cost-sharing and so on--is compatible with these requirements is not an issue I want to address directly here, however.

Second, there are important resource allocation implications of the fair equality of opportunity approach. Access

to a given health care system does not guarantee that risk of
encountering health and opportunity impairments is equitably
distributed. Extensive preventive measures, including environmental and safety measures, are important on this view if
risk and not just treatment is to be equitably distributed.
But such considerations involve important allocation decisions, and resources--including manpower--must be provided.
Another relevant kind of allocation decision concerns the
meeting of unmet needs by creating new or expanded categories of services--e.g. gerontological specialization is
formally recognized in Great Britain but not the US. So
there is a social obligation to channel medical professionals
into delivery settings where they are most needed. Yet
another allocational issue highlighted by this analysis concerns the relative attention paid to 'purely medical' efforts
to restore normal functioning and the 'social support' that
might be required to compensate for lost functioning and
the 'social support' that might be required to compensate for
lost functioning when medical intervention is no longer
feasible. The fair equality of opportunity principle suggests,
I believe, that much underprovided social support--e.g.
seeing-eye dogs for the blind--is functionally comparable to
the more glamorous (and profitable) medical services and
should be given greater emphasis.

If there are these--and other--distributive implications
of the fair equality of opportunity approach I have sketched,
and if we can assume a moderate scarcity of resources, then
it is safe to conclude that resources will not be adequate
to maximizing absolute quality for all patients. Such constraints can be viewed as 'budget ceilings' imposed at a
macro allocation level. These reflect the relative importance of different diseases and the health care needs they
generate. What this amounts to, then, is the claim that
what Donabedian calls "social costs" (assuming minimal cost-
sharing) must play a role in at least macro-allocation
decisions (Donabedian, 1979, p. 283-4).

How does this argument affect the view I sketched
earlier of the role of the physician in the pursuit of
absolute quality? I think it does not force us to abandon
that model but only to qualify it. It suggests that the
physician has the task of advising the patient about the
best treatment package, the one with the greatest absolute
quality, available under the resource constraints imposed
by considerations of justice. The physician remains in this

way primarily the agent of the patient, though he operates under some social constraints. Still, he does not have to import into his own case by case decision-making inferences from general social principles that, at another level, determine macro-allocations. Such an arrangement need not jeopardize patient confidence in the physician. Moreover, the patient's entitlements to health care services are constrained by considerations of justice. But the constraints are not ones he should see the physician as having imposed. It is not the physician who here implicitly puts a price on the patient's life.

It may seem to some that a system which permits the pursuit of maximal absolute quality in the micro-situation is less intrusive than the one I sketch. More to the point, by refusing to put a price on life, it may seem to be morally preferable. But I think this is an illusion. Such a system would still require rationing in some other way-- e.g. by ability to pay for health care--assuming resources are not infinite. For those who cannot gain access to health care services because they cannot afford them, the implicit price on life is quite low. This point aside, I think the 'ability to pay' rationing system violates fundamental requirements of justice bearing on the fair distribution of health care resources and so constitutes a greater moral evil than the need to place a price on life.

It should be obvious from my sketch of a theory of distributive justice for health care that I am not accepting "efficiency" considerations alone as the basis for macro allocation decisions. What may be called equity considerations play the key role. But there is plenty of room, within the approach I sketch, to insert cost-benefit and cost-effectiveness methodology, for within the constraints justice imposes on our allocations, we want to be cost-effective. Still, and this is an important point, it is not just the demands of efficiency that lead us to "put a price on life" in conditions of moderate scarcity; it is the demands of justice itself. Pricing life is not simply the result of worshipping the almighty buck but is something forced on us if we aspire to be just in distributing limited resources.

If we are going to allow room for cost-benefit and cost-effectiveness analyses, then we must address some specific ethical issues raised by their use. Before turning to the use of cost-effectiveness analysis in the Neuhauser-Lewicki study, I would like to make a few brief remarks about cost-benefit analysis since it is more likely to be thought a methdology usable in overall macro-allocation decision making.

We should note right away that cost-benefit analysis, because it attempts to convert all benefits into monetary units, faces problems that cost-effectiveness analysis, of the sort used in our Neuhauser and Lewicki case study, does not face. The apparent advantage of attempting such a monetary conversion is that it allows one to compare otherwise quite different packages of benefits. The price paid for the advantage is that serious equity questions arise about the three main methodologies available for converting life-extending services into dollar benefits. For example, the attempt to calculate 'earning streams' generated by a life-extending technology--the so called 'productivity measure'--faces standard objections that it reflects the inequities of wage differences by social class, race, and sex and age. The attempt to 'price life' by deriving dollar valuations implicit in public policy programs already in operation faces the objection that very different values are implicit in different areas of public policy. Finally, the approach that seems to have the best theoretical rationale, the 'willingness-to-pay' standard, raises other difficulties (Mishan, E.J., 1969, 1971, 1976; Schelling, 1968; Acton, 1976; Bayles, 1978). It is quite difficult to derive meaningful estimates of willingness-to-pay for the reduction in risk to life that are controlled for biases induced by initial income inequalities. But even if one can accomplish such a derivation, willingness to pay estimates are still subject to various kinds of biasing. Cancer phobia, for example, might lead to inflated 'willingness-to pay' figures, inflated, that is, relative to more objective estimates of the importance of reducing the risk of cancer relative to other conditions. One might hope for some more objective basis, one not so open to subjective biases, for assessing the relative importance of reducing risks for different disease conditions. Elsewhere, I have suggested that the effects of different conditions on opportunity ranges may provide an objective corrective to willingess to pay measures.

My own view is that these methodological difficulties--with their attendant ethical worries--reinforce the view that cost-benefit analysis is no substitute for a theory of distributive justice that addresses resource allocation problems. And this conclusion is further reinforced when we remember that at best cost-benefit analysis tells us that a policy option yields a certain potential pareto improvement, or allows us to compare the potential pareto improvements of different options. But the fact that a potential pareto improvement is present tells us nothing about how the gain is to be distributed, and so leaves equity problems lurking in the wings again.

Fortunately, the Neuhauser and Lewicki cost-effectiveness study of the stool guaiac screening procedure for colon cancer inherits few of these problems facing cost-benefit analysis in general. In it, all benefits are expressed as the detection of colon cancer in a screened patient. The benefits of saving a life or extending it do not have to be converted into dollars. What is pointed out is the cost-variation implicit in different screening procedures for the delivery of a common benefit--the detection of a colon cancer. We learn that the marginal cost of detecting a cancer on the sixth guaiac test is over $47 million (and $4.7 million on the fifth test). How much is the extra reduction in risk worth? (The sixth test costs an extra $13,190 for the discovery of .0003 cases in a population of 10,000 with an incidence of 72, given a test sensitivity of almost 92%). (Neuhauser & Lewicki, 1973, p. 227).[1] Here the methodology is posing a question to us without providing an answer. As we shall see, answering it is quite difficult without being able to make a variety of simplifying assumptions.

Consider the following argument someone might make. Suppose we propose a cut-off after the 5th test. Then it seems that the implicit valuation we are putting on the detection of a colon cancer is no more than $4.7 million. But this valuation is clearly less than we are willing to spend to save lives in some other contexts--e.g. the safety devices that surround an air force pilot. Card and Mooney cite an example of a building code change in Great Britain, following the collapse of an apartment building, which was calculated to place an implicit value of ₤20 million on a life saved (Card and Mooney, 1977). Even allowing for the

[1]It is important to note that these figures assume no intermittent bleeding and thus a roughly equal probability of bleeding in each stool sample. Some have challenged this assumption on medical grounds, but I will here ignore these objections for the sake of argument.

fluctuation of the dollar, this figure is comparable to the marginal cost per cancer detected of the 6th stool guaiac. So cutting off screening at the 5th test seriously under-values life compared to these other valuations.

There are problems with this argument. For one thing, there are also public policies in which the implicit value placed on saving a life is far less than $4.7 million. Card and Mooney suggest the National Health Service decision not to put safety caps on prescription bottles implicitly placed a maximum value on the life of a child of Ł1,000. Why pick the higher 'value of life' figure? For another, there may be reasons that justify the high expenditure in one setting-- e.g. the pilot example--which do not apply in the health care setting. But a more important point can be brought out by asking "What will be done with the money saved if the screening procedure is stopped with five guaiacs?" If the money is redistributed to yield more efficient saving of lives in the health care system, that might seem a worth-while goal. If the money will simply yield higher profits for insurance company investors, that might seem a less worthwhile goal. But before one knows just what to do with Neuhauser-Lewicki data, we have to have some idea what al-ternative uses there are for the resources. But having a reasonable idea about such alternatives requires adopting a macro-allocational perspective.

To see what I mean, consider the problem from the per-spective of the micro setting--I am the patient and I happen to have read the Neuhauser-Lewicki paper. From my point of view, I say, "Well, it's only $1 for the extra test and I am sufficiently afraid of cancer and sufficiently risk-aversive that it is worth it to me to have the extra test." I might say this whether or not I paid the $1 out of pocket (I might feel quite differently about a far more expensive test pro-ducing comparable risk reduction/dollar, which only goes to show how subjective--and how income sensitive--some of the willingness to pay estimates we make may be). My physician might agree with my preference--for he too might place a value on my gaining reassurance. And in any case, neither he nor I can be sure that the dollar not spent will be rein-vested elsewhere with greater effect. From the micro-perspective, the problem seems all too easy to solve. Yet, as Neuhauser and Lewicki point out in another paper, de-ciding to go to six guaiacs buys freedom from fear at a marginal cost of $327,547 per 1 percent reduction in the probability of having silent cancer (Neuhauser and Lewicki, 1976, p. 186). If we can imagine that my cancer phobia and my inability to handle calculations about low probabilities are not atypical, and that most people will act similarly, then leaving the problem to micro-decision making might force the macro-expenditure on the 6th stool guaiac. In a context of resource scarcity, it may not only be inefficient but inequitable to refuse to set a macro policy on the question.

My discussion does not tell us just what to do with the Neuhauser-Lewicki data. We do not have enough information to act on that data. In the absence of comparative data for a broad range of other procedures, in the absence of some assurance that a utilization decision about the 6th stool guaiac will be translated, somewhere along the line, into more efficient and more equitable utilization decisions elsewhere in the system, we at best have some reason to think we can do better than use a 6th guaiac. In any case, we would have to face the problem about where the decision should be taken. Should the American Cancer Society protocol be revised--so that it is seen as "good medicine" simply to do five or four tests? Should the decision be made by third-party payers--who might refuse to reimburse for more than four or five guaiacs? Should the decision be made by the hospital or HMO--where greater control over alternative uses of the money saved may be present? Or should we see the individual physician as the person responsible for introducing some cost-effectiveness calculations into his estimate of what counts as "good medical care"--despite the fact that he may be deviating from ACS protocols in doing so?

REFERENCES

Acton, JP (1976). Measuring the monetary value of life-saving programs. Law and Contemporary Problems XL:4, 46-72.
Bayles, M (1978). The price of life. Ethics 89:1, 20-34.
Card, W and Mooney, GH (1977). What is the monetary value of a human life? Brit Med J 2:1627-1629.
Donabedian, A (1979). The quality of medical care: a concept in search of a definition. J Fam Practice 9:2, 277-284.
Mishan, EJ (1969). "Welfare Economics: An Assessment." North Holland.

Mishan, EJ (1971). Evaluation of life and limb: a theoretical approach. J Polit Econ 79:4, 687-705.

Mishan, EJ (1976). "Cost-Benefit Analysis." Praeger.

Neuhauser, D and Lewicki, AM (1973). What do we gain from the sixth stool guaiac? NEJM 293:5, 226-228.

Neuhauser, D and Lewicki, AM (1976). National Health Insurance and the sixth stool guaiac. Policy Analysis 2:2, 175-196.

Rawls, J (1971). "A Theory of Justice." Cambridge: Harvard. §14.

Schelling, T (1968). The life you save may be your own. In Chase, SB (ed) "Problems in Public Policy Expenditure Analysis." Washington, D.C.:Brookings.

Rights and Responsibilities in Modern Medicine: The Second
Volume in a Series on Ethics, Humanism, and Medicine: 171—176
© 1981 Alan R. Liss, Inc., 150 Fifth Avenue, New York, NY 10011

COST EFFECTIVENESS AND PATIENT WELFARE

Meredith Eiker, M.P.H. and John N. Sheagren

V.A. Medical Center and University of Michigan

Ann Arbor, Michigan

The title of this discussion is "Cost Effectiveness and
Patient Welfare." Perhaps the best place to start is with
some definitions and assumptions. Looking first at "cost,"
one needs to think in terms, obviously, of dollars or economic considerations. Equally important, however, is the
awareness that the costs associated with health care may
also be identified in terms of social, political, and ethical considerations. Further, costs must be assigned not
only to the delivery of medical care, but also to any decision not to provide some component or other of medical care.

In talking about "effectiveness," care must be taken
not to confuse effectiveness with efficiency or efficacy or
with such other cost issues as cost containment. Specifically, "efficacy" refers to that which has the power to produce desired results; for instance, with the choice of a
drug such as an antibiotic. One cannot really sensibly talk
about "cost efficacy" because the "cost" is not the thing
which produces the result.

"Efficiency" has to do with the ability to produce the
desired result with the minimum effort, expense, or waste
and relates to skill and economy of energy. Taking a decision, for instance, that nafcillin is the most efficacious
drug to use in the treatment of a given infectious disease,
one is left with the further decision of how to administer
the drug. If the drug is administered intravenously, then
more nursing resources may be used though the length of the
hospital stay may be decreased. On the other hand, one might
choose to administer the drug intramuscularly or orally,

thereby decreasing nursing time but perhaps increasing the length of the course of therepy.

"Effectiveness" has to do with the impact of the result, the size of the bang in relation to the size of the buck. One can be effective without necessarily being efficient and without using the most efficacious means.

No definition of "patient" appears to be necessary; however, worth mentioning is the fact that "welfare," specifically patient welfare, can mean a lot of things. Some people, quite frankly, are better off dead.

Discussions such as this one have arisen because of some intrinsic confusion over these definitions. The confusion is not in the grammar or semantics, but rather in the application of these terms to the health care industry. Generally, society is concerned with economic costs and people tend to take the pie slices and bar graphs and insurance premiums and conclude that health care is too expensive. Indeed, the health care industry is the third largest industry in the United States today behind agriculture and construction. More than 10 per cent of the United States Gross National Product goes to health care and that percentage is growing. Where will the growth end? At 12 per cent? 15 per cent? 25 per cent?

Right here, when the discussion begins to turn to a limit to the growth of the health care industry, a fundamental value judgement is made: That is, that health care should not consume a growing portion of the nation's resources. That value judgement implies that providers and consumers of health care should make adjustments to assure that the industry does not proliferate outside of whatever the growth -- and cost -- boundaries are.

In order to accomplish the objective of containing growth, so as to accomplish the objective of containing dollar costs, society looks to the health care industry and urges what are essentially "self" controls. For instance, the industry is expected to reduce excess bed capacity, restrict the purchase of high technology items such as CT scanners which are prone to under-utilization, eliminate unnecessary tests and surgeries, become more efficient, etc. Society expects and demands, however, that all of this will be done by physicians and administrators and other health

care professionals without any impact on the availability
and accessibility of health care and certainly without any
reduction in the quality of health care.

Society seems to assume that finite resources will have
an infinite ability to meet all of the health care needs and
most of the health care demands. Even if one is not so naive
as to assume that finite resources can be expanded infinitely, the individual does frequently assume that the impact
of economic cost considerations will not enter directly into
individual episodes of care. One expects the issues and
impacts to remain macro -- system oriented -- concerns and
not micro -- individualized -- confrontations.

Why does society want to limit the health care industry's growth? Who will decide that limit and how will the
decisions be made? Who will implement the limit, place the
controls? Why does society expect the health care industry
to be self-limiting, self-regulating? Why does society think
that this can all be accomplished at a macro, or system,
level when, in fact, health care is by definition personal
and individual? Clearly, the health care industry is not
like the construction industry where in housing for instance,
the needs and demands equate to so many units of shelter; or
like the agriculture industry where the units are so many
tomatoes and carrots.

The health care industry, or as some experts are now
choosing to call it, the "sickness" care industry, finds
itself today facing tough economic choices. These are
choices, however, which are not strictly economic at all,
but are rather ethical and moral choices which society simply
does not want to acknowledge as such and which society is
more comfortable with when they are disguised as economic
or cost related. Further, by misrepresenting these issues
as economic, society has been able to "pass the buck" and
responsibilities for them to a small group of people: specifically, to the supposed health care industry experts, the
health care providers themselves, and to the government
and some innocent economists.

Here again, one might argue that responsibilities for
these issues lies with society, massively and collectively,
and that these issues are related to social goals and objectives, social values, and social outcomes. This confusion
of social and ethical and moral and political and economic

issues in health care, as long as it persists, belies what for many is a fundamental confusion in our society at large -- a confusion which precludes society from setting rational national health care priorities.

The literature, the experts speaking today, confirm that nothing will be added to the health status of anyone or to the quality of life of anyone by adding dollars to the health care industry. The industry has not yet learned to use well all the tools and knowledge already available. Unrealistic expectations prevail as to what health care can do for the individual.

One might ask what objectives the individual holds personally for the health care industry. Prevention? Cure? Comfort? Improvement in the quality of life? Maintenance of health? Maintenance of life? Restoration of health? As long as the confusion around desired objectives and outcomes exists, the health care professionals cannot possibly figure out the mix of inputs.

Society has left the decision making to the supposed experts, to health care professionals. For instance, who really decides in the choice between comfort and cure? And if the decision is comfort, pain relief for the terminal cancer patient, then how much comfort? Addicting pain medications or palliative surgery to prolong life just a little bit? Who is really monitoring the directions of preventive medicine? Are clean air standards to be advocated as vigorously as immunizations? A lot of medicine is practiced to relieve physician anxiety because physicians do not have clear directives from society. Physicians are not taught to practice social or ethical or political or economic medicine, they are taught to practice scientific medicine, to rely on technology.

Physicians are asked daily to make decisions about the value of an individual human life -- who to triage out of the intensive care unit for instance. How does the physician make that decision? What social, ethical, political, and economic guidance does he/she have?

Card and Mooney suggest three approaches related to the valuation of life in what they call the "medicopolitical system."[1] First, they suggest that a human life might be valued according to the individual's productive capacity.

The individual's productivity is calculated in terms of estimated earnings, years of participation in the work force, support of family members, etc. Implied, however, in this methodology is the assumption that one of the primary objectives of the health care industry is to add to the productive capacity of the nation.

The second approach to the valuation of human life as suggested by Card and Mooney relates to general implicit values such as those which arise with social policy decisions. Here, social and political decision-making may result in a determination not to allocate resources to a life-saving policy. These decisions are most clearly evident in such areas as occupational health, environmental protection, and automobile safety. The choice of not providing a health-enhancing benefit implies that the return on saving a life is less than the cost of saving the life. If fifteen lives will be saved by a fifteen million dollar alteration to a factory, than the value of a single life is estimated at one million dollars. Is one life worth a million dollars?

The third approach for valuating a human life as described by Card and Mooney deals with the individual's values. This determination focuses on the value placed on reducing the risk of death rather than on the absolute value of the human life. It assumes that the individual will make health-enhancing choices such as opting for not smoking and more exercise. The individual then valuates his own life, measurable in terms of risk-reducing behavior changes.

The key point here appears to be that the individual values his life and the lives of others differently at different times. For instance, the individual seems to be willing to invest more when he or she is sick than when well. Following a heart attack, the incentive to quit smoking is greater. Or, in another example, no one was interested in buying a Pinto which cost $10,000 but quite a few people were indignant when $3,500 Pintos were found to have vulnerable gas tanks and a few people died.

The relationship of cost effectiveness and patient welfare seems to depend to a great extent on contextual factors. Clean air standards may or may not be viewed as cost effective until 10 per cent of the population deve-

lops emphysema. Cost effectiveness should not, and cannot
in fact, be an attainable goal of the health care system
until the parameters of patient welfare are defined. The
dilemma appears to be that of whether to define cost effectiveness in terms of patient welfare or patient welfare in
terms of cost effectiveness. Neither set of definitions,
however, is likely to be strictly economic, though the
tendency of late has been to reduce the health care system
to a series of economic choices and trade-offs. Many
health care professionals are tiring of talking about cost
effectiveness in health care and about their responsibilities for economic costs without also talking about the
ethical, social, moral, and political costs of health
care and the broad societal responsibilities for those
costs.

A very simple system for eliminating the cost questions might be suggested, particularly if no one is willing
to deal with these broader issues. The nation talks daily
about rationing other scarce, expensive resources. Why
not talk about rationing health care? The rationing would
not be done by physicians or by administrators but rather
by individuals themselves. Everyone would get a health
care ticket: so many dollars at birth or so many dollars
per year. Use of the ticket would be limited to the individual and would be non-negotiable on the open market. The
individual would become a true consumer of health care and
the hospital or clinic would become just another super-
market selling goods at retail prices. The consumer could
choose among prevention, cure (if it's in stock), comfort,
lab tests, operations, whatever. This would be a nice,
easy, controllable, and amoral system -- a micro system
fully personalized and individualized. It would also pass
the buck -- right back where it belongs, in society's lap.

REFERENCES

1. Card WI, Mooney GH (1977). What is the monetary value
of a human life? Brit Med J 2;1627.

DISCUSSION SUMMARY: COST EFFECTIVENESS AND PATIENT WELFARE

Marc D. Basson

Director, CEHM
University of Michigan
Ann Arbor, Michigan

Many of the participants brought up concerns outside the
specific issues aimed at by the questions at the end of the
case but which were nonetheless valid. Thus, several pointed
out that the "cost-effectiveness" of a decision on this case
depended on where the money would go if not spent on stool
guaiacs. (Would insurance companies donate it for a public
health education plan? Would they pocket the extra money as
a profit? Would they pass the savings back down to the patients?) "We need a guarantee," one group concluded, "that if
we are cost-effective as physicians, then the money will be
used fairly as part of a health care reallocation." Others
questioned the validity of the statistics or medical details
of the case.

The basic decisions which all groups attempted to make
were: (1) How many stool guaiacs would you want as a patient
eligible for screening? (2) How many stool guaiacs would you
perform as a physician? Most said that they would probably
want two or three tests themselves, although several said that
they would request a full series of six because they were
afraid of cancer. These people pointed out that in addition
to protection from cancer, they would be buying an additional
increment of security with the extra tests: the knowledge
that they were healthy.

The question of how many tests the physician ought to
perform was more controversial. The group that had insisted
on (and not received) guarantees as to how the money saved
would be spent voted to recommend a six test series to the
physician. About 10 percent refused to name a number of tests,

justifying their refusal with one participant's argument that "we need to keep medicine on the micro level, regardless of cost, since that is the essence of the art of medicine."

The rest of the participants almost unanimously voted to do only one test for routine screening, reasoning that the money could be better used elsewhere and that the physician was obliged to see that it was so used. This obligation, they felt, stemmed from the fact that society at large pays for each person's individual medical expenses through health insurance. Thus, other third parties enter into the previously dyadic doctor-patient relationship because they have paid for the medical care. If the patient specifically requested more than one test, most were willing to do this provided the patient was willing to pay for the extra tests himself rather than through his insurance.

Interestingly, although almost all the groups were able to arrive at a consensus on the number of tests they would routinely do, none were willing to explicitly name the monetary value they would place on a human life. Many stated that a specific figure was unnecessary while others felt that "the chance of saving a human life is not worth forty seven million dollars, but my human life is very valuable and no worth can ever be set on it."

INTRODUCTION: RATIONAL SUICIDE

Marc D. Basson

Director, CEHM
University of Michigan
Ann Arbor, Michigan

Suicide is a difficult issue for anyone to deal with,
as it is inextricably bound up in the despair of the victim
and the self-recriminations of the survivors who failed to
help. It is especially troubling to physicians who dedicate
themselves to keeping patients alive. Indeed, some doctors
will still admit if pressed that they consider rational
suicide impossible since deliberately seeking one's death is
insane. Many others will admit in principle that some
patient's wish to die might conceivably be rational but doubt
that they will ever encounter such a patient. It is ironic
that the same medical technology that permits these doctors
to dedicate themselves to prolonging life has created a new
class of patients: diagnosed, perhaps palliated, but uncured
and alive, who might seek death.

The fundamental ethical issues implicit in our treatment
of such patients and the possibilities of euthanasia for them
can often be sidestepped by denying the patient's competence
to request or give an informed consent to his death. The
case of rational suicide sharpens our focus since no such
evasion is possible. Discussion of such hard cases is therefore doubly valuable for moral introspection.

Each of the two speakers on this topic lays out an
extreme position, thoughtfully developed from fundamental
ethical assumptions clearly not shared by the other speaker.
The reader who wishes to adopt a more moderate stance may
learn much from trying to meet the challenges each extremist
offers.

Stanley Hauerwas's philosophy is unabashedly religious in both flavor and content. He takes the moral wrongness of suicide to be unquestionable, while freely conceding that at least some morally wrong suicides may seem rationally indicated. His willingness to ignore evasive quibbles about the impossibility of rational suicide is impressive.

Hauerwas recognizes that if a rational suicide is morally wrong, this must be because of something or someone external to the would-be suicide. Others have pointed to unfulfilled obligations to fellow-men or to the harm to the survivors as reasons against suicide. Hauerwas's religious background enables him to give a different answer. God, Hauerwas says, has given us our lives (or at least lent them to us?) and we therefore have an obligation to God to refrain from suicide. Hauerwas notes that he is using the "language of gift" in this discussion, but where more secular philosophies might hesitate to infer obligation from an unsolicited gift, Hauerwas imbues his language of gift with an overtone of commandment.

Jerome Motto is a psychiatrist who has done a great deal of work in suicide counselling and prevention. He, too, begins with the premise that some suicides are rational. He goes on to state as a second basic premise that at least some of these suicides are morally permissible. The major thrust of his paper is advice as to how the counsellor and patient together can decide whether the proposed suicide is indeed one of the permissible ones.

Along the way, Motto makes several interesting statements. He urges that all alternatives to suicide be explored and that the patient "see all the facts clearly." However, Motto also notes that he would accept a patient's evaluation of the situation even if it seemed wrong "if it is the best judgment the patient is capable of exercising." Motto does not elaborate on this thought, but one must wonder just how far he is prepared to go in his rejection of paternalism. If the patient is suffering from a documented and intractable mental or emotional disorder which will always alter his judgment, would Motto still accept this? (A case could be made for such acceptance. The patient might say that he would rather be dead that continue to be depressed.)

Motto also defines an ethical obligation to tell the patient's family that the patient is contemplating suicide,

even if the patient objects. It is not clear how he recon-
ciles this seemingly paternalistic view with the permissive
moral principles he expresses in the rest of his paper. The
issue of confidentiality in psychiatry is a tricky one.

Our case for this topic involves a man newly diagnosed
as having Huntington's Chorea. It has elements that Motto
might consider important, such as the possible ambivalence
demonstrated by the patient's consulting a psychiatrist and
then contemplating suicide in his house. For Hauerwas, of
course, the only important element is that the patient has
a God-given life or soul. There are also a number of other
considerations buried in the case, such as the patient's
family obligations and the question of whether it would be
rational to wait until the disease progresses to the point
of incapacitation. Additional questions for the reader to
consider involve the proper role of the bystander. May the
patient's wife interfere because she is his wife or because
she is Catholic and believes suicide to be morally wrong?
How ought doctors to behave towards a would-be suicide?
Do their professional ethics prohibit cooperation? Do they
mandate interference? Is there a special set of rules for
"emergency room ethics" in which doctors must save lives first
and ask questions later? The case, like the issue, is
complicated. There is much to learn from the effort to un-
tangle both.

Rights and Responsibilities in Modern Medicine: The Second
Volume in a Series on Ethics, Humanism, and Medicine: 183–184
© 1981 Alan R. Liss, Inc., 150 Fifth Avenue, New York, NY 10011

THE RATIONAL SUICIDE

Case for Discussion

Huntington's chorea has been described as "the most horrible of neurologic disorders." There are two major symptoms of Huntington's chorea. The first is "choreiform movements," rapid uncontrollable twitchings and contortions of the voluntary muscles of the face and hands, and later of the trunk and extremities as well. The second is a progressive dementia, deterioration of the victim's memory and higher intellectual function. Either class of symptoms may precede the other by up to several years and some patients experience a rapid worsening while others may remain only mildly symptomatic for some years. The dementia is irreversible and only slight amelioration of the chorea is obtainable with current medical therapy. The disease generally appears in the third or fourth decade of life, and despite the variation in rate of progression its course is always an inexorable worsening of symptoms, with death ensuing in about ten years.

The disease is inherited as an autosomal dominant. This means that every child of an affected parent has a fifty percent chance of having the disease. Since it appears late in life and there is no way to predict who will develop it, there is no shortage of children of diseased parents. However, as these children grow up, their father or mother suffers from and is killed by Huntington's chorea and they must live with the knowledge that it may afflict them as well. There is a significantly higher incidence of alcoholism, mental illness and juvenile delinquency among these children.

John Kelsey is a thirty-two-year-old lawyer whose

mother died from Huntington's chorea. He is married and has one child, a three year old son resulting from a contraception failure. (His wife is Catholic and they agreed not to have an abortion.) John is productively employed but drinks five or six martinis per day and has been seeing a psychiatrist for several years for intermittent bouts of depression. Always deeply anxious about the possibility of developing Huntington's chorea, he has many times told his wife, his psychiatrist and close friends that he would rather die than have to live as he remembers his mother.

He noticed the onset of facial twitching three months ago but did not mention it to anyone. He then consulted two neurologists each of whom independently diagnosed his problem as Huntington's.

Three days ago he revealed this to his psychiatrist and asked him for something with which to commit suicide. The psychiatrist was sympathetic but advised John that he could not do this. Well aware of the law that permitted his involuntary committment if deemed dangerous to himself, John convinced his psychiatrist that he was not planning any immediate action. He then went home, wrote a long letter explaining his reasons for action, pinned it to his shirt, and swallowed the remaining tablets in his bottle of anti-depressant medication. He was found shortly thereafter by his wife and rushed to the hospital unconscious, with his letter still pinned to his shirt. The letter also expressed John's refusal of medical treatment for poisoning.

Is suicide ever morally permissible? If not, is it ever morally permissible to help someone kill himself? To allow him to do so?

Would it have been morally permissible for the psychiatrist (who was firmly convinced that John was fully rational) to have written the requested prescription? Given that events transpired as above, what should the emergency room physician do? Would it be wrong to pump John's stomach in the emergency room? To attempt to resuscitate him if his heart stopped? What bearing, if any, do the existence and desires of John's wife and son have on these questions?

Rights and Responsibilities in Modern Medicine: The Second
Volume in a Series on Ethics, Humanism, and Medicine: 185—199
© 1981 Alan R. Liss, Inc.,150 Fifth Avenue, New York, NY 10011

RATIONAL SUICIDE AND REASONS FOR LIVING

Stanley Hauerwas
University of Notre Dame
Notre Dame, Indiana

1. SUICIDE AND THE ETHICS OF AUTONOMY

There is a peculiar ambiguity concerning the morality of
suicide in our society. Our commitment to the autonomy of
the individual at least implies that suicide may not only be
rational, but a "right."[1] Yet many continue to believe that
anyone attempting suicide must be sick and therefore prevented
from killing themselves. This ambiguity makes us hesitant
even to analyze the morality of suicide because we fear we may
discover that our society lacks any coherent moral policy or
basis for preventing suicide.

Therefore the very idea of "rational suicide" is a bit
threatening. We must all feel a slight twinge of concern
about the book soon to be published by the British Voluntary
Euthanasia Society that describes the various painless and
foolproof methods of suicide. But it is by no means clear why
we feel uncomfortable about having this kind of book widely
distributed. As Nicholas Reed, the general secretary of the
Society, suggests: suicide is "more and more seen as an acceptable way for a life to end, vastly preferable to some long,
slow, painful death. We're simply helping in the fight for
another human right--the right to die" (New York Times, 1980:
A18).

[1]For example Beauchamp and Childress (1979:90) suggest,
"If the principle of autonomy is strongly relied upon for the
justification of suicide, then it would seem that there is a
right to commit suicide, so long as a person acts autonomously
and does not seriously affect the interests of others."

We think there must be something wrong with this, but we are not sure what. I suspect our unease about these matters is part of the reason we wish to deny the existence of rational or autonomous suicide. If all potential suicides can be declared ill by definition then we can prevent them ironically because the agent lacks autonomy. Therefore we intervene to prevent suicides in the name of autonomy which, if we were consistent, should require us to consider suicide a permissible moral act.

Once I was a participant in a seminar in medical ethics at one of our most prestigious medical schools. I was there to speak about suicide, but the week before the seminar had considered abortion. At that time I was told by these beginning medical students they decided it was their responsibility to perform an abortion if a woman requested it because a woman has the right to determine what she should do with her body--a ethical conclusion that they felt clearly justified on grounds of protecting the autonomy of the patient. Moreover this position, they argued, was appropriate if the professional dominance and paternalism of the medical profession was to be broken.

However, I asked them what they would do if they were attending in the Emergency Room and someone was brought in with slashed wrists with a suicide note pinned to their shirt front. First of all would they take the time to read the note to discover the state of the patient? Secondly would they say this is clearly not a medical matter and refuse to accept the patient? Or would they immediately begin to save the person's life? With the same unanimity concerning their responsibility to perform abortion they felt they must immediately begin trying to save the person's life.

The reason they gave to justify their intervention was that anyone taking their life must surely be sick. But it was not clear what kind of "sickness" was under consideration unless we define life itself as some kind of syndrome. Failing to make the case that all suicides must be sick they then suggested they must act to save such a person's life because it was their responsibility as doctors. But again I pressed them on what right they had to impose their role-related responsibilities on those who did not seek their services and, in fact, had clearly tried to avoid coming in contact with them. They then appealed to experience, citing cases when people have recovered from suicide attempts only to be thankful they had been helped. But again such appeals are not convincing since we can also point to the many who are not happy about being saved and soon make another attempt.

Our discussion began to be more and more frustrating for all involved, so a compromise was suggested. These future physicians felt the only solution was when a suicide came to the Emergency Room the first time the doctor's responsibility must always be to save their life. However if they came in a second time they could be allowed to die. That kind of solution, however, is not only morally unsatisfactory, but pragmatically difficult to institutionalize. What happens if each time the person is brought to the hospital they get a different physician?

I have told this story because I think it nicely illustrates the kind of difficulties we feel when we try to get a moral handle on suicide. We feel that Beauchamp and Childress are right that if a suicide is genuinely autonomous and there is no powerful utilitarian reasons for "reasons of human worth and dignity standing in the way, then we ought to allow the person to commit suicide, because we would otherwise be violating the person's autonomy" (Beauchamp, Childress, 1979:93).

However I want to suggest that this way of putting the matter, while completely consistent with an ethics of autonomy, is also deeply misleading. It is misleading not only because it reveals the insufficiency of autonomy either as a basis or ideal for the moral life (Bergmann, 1977; Dworkin, 1978) but also it simply fails to provide an appropriate account of why any of us decide or should decide to stay alive. Indeed it is odd even to think of our willingness to live as a decision. For example Beauchamp and Childress do not explain how anyone could take account of <u>all</u> relevant variables and future possibilities in considering suicide. Indeed that seems an odd condition for if we required it of even our most important decisions it would stop us from acting at all.

Yet by challenging this account I want clearly to distinguish my position from those who are intent to deny the possibility of rational suicide. I think that suicide can be and often is a rational decision of an "autonomous" agent, but I do not therefore think it is justified. It is extremely interesting, for example, that Augustine did not claim that suicide was irrational in criticizing the Stoic acceptance and even recommendation of suicide. Rather he pointed out that their acceptance of suicide belied their own understanding of the relation between evil and happiness and how a wise man thus should deal with adversity. Though the quote is long I think it worth providing the full text. Augustine says,

> There is a mighty force in the evils which compel a man, and, according to those philosophers, even a wise man, to rob himself of his existence as a man; although they say, and say with truth, that the first and greatest utterance of nature, as we may call it, is that a man should be reconciled to himself and for that reason should naturally shun death--that he should be his own friend, in that he should emphatically desire to continue as a living being and to remain alive in this combination of body and soul, and that this should be his aim. There is a mighty force in those evils which overpower this natural feeling which makes us employ all our strength in our endeavor to avoid death--which defeat this feeling so utterly that what was shunned is now wished and longed for, and, if it cannot come to him from some other source, is inflicted on a man by himself. There is a mighty force in those evils which make Fortitude a murderer--if indeed she is still to be called fortitude when she is so utterly vanquished by those evils that she not only cannot by her endurance keep guard over the man she has undertaken to govern and protect, but is herself compelled to go so far as to kill him. The wise man ought, indeed, to endure even death with a steadfastness, but a death that comes to him from outside himself. Whereas if he is compelled, as those philosophers say, to inflict it on himself, they must surely admit that these are not only evils, but intolerable evils, when they compel him to commit this crime.
>
> It follows from this that the life weighed down by such great and grievous ills, or at the mercy of such chances, would never be called happy, if the men who so term it, and who, when overcome by the growing weights of ills, surrender to adversity incompassing their own

death--if these people would bring themselves to
surrender to the truth, when overcome by sound
reasoning, in their quest for the happy life, and
would give up supposing that the ultimate, Supreme
God is something to be enjoyed by them in this
condition of morality (1977:856-857).

The question is not, therefore, the question of whether
suicide is "rational," Augustine knew well that the Stoics
could provide outstanding examples of cool, unemotional, and
rational suicide. He rather asks what kind of blessedness
we should expect out of life. For Augustine the Stoic approval of suicide was an indication of the insufficient
account they provided about what human existence should be
about--namely they failed to see that the only happiness
worth desiring is that which came from friendship with the
true God. "Yet" he says, "these philosophers refuse to believe in this blessedness because they do not see it; and so
they attempt to fabricate for themselves an utterly delusive
happiness by means of a virtue whose falsity is in proportion to its arrogance" (Augustine, 1977:857).[2] So the issue,
if Augustine is right as I believe him to be, is how suicide
is understood within a conception of life we think good and
worthy.

2. THE GRAMMAR OF SUICIDE

Before developing this line of reasoning, however, it
should be pointed out that the discussion to this point has
been trading on the assumption that we know what suicide is.

[2]Earlier Augustine had argued, "There were famous heroes
who, though by the laws of war they could do violence to a
conquered enemy, refuse to do violence to themselves when
conquered; though they had not the slightest fear of death,
they choose to endure the enemys domination rather than put
themselves to death. They were fighting for their earthly
country; but the Gods they worshipped were false; but their
worship was genuine and they faithfully kept their oaths.
Christians worship the true God and they yearn for a heavenly
country; will they not have more reason to refrain from the
crime of suicide, if God's providence subjects them for a
time to their enemies for their probation or reformation.
Their God does not abandon them in that humiliation, for he
came from on high so humbly for their sake" (1977:35-36).

Yet that is simply not the case. For as Beauchamp and Childress suggest, definitions of suicide such as "an intentionally caused self-destruction not forced by the action of another person" are not nearly as unambiguous as they may at first seem. For example they point out when persons suffering from a terminal illness or mortal injury allow their death to occur we find ourselves reluctant to call that act "suicide," but if persons with a terminal illness take their life by active means we do refer to that act as one of suicide. Yet to only describe those acts that involved a direct action as suicide is misleading since we are not sure how we should describe cases where "a patient with a terminal condition might easily avoid dying for a long time but might choose to end his life immediately by not taking cheap and painless medication" (Beauchamp, Childress, 1974:86).

Beauchamp and Childress suggest the reason we have difficulty deciding the meaning of suicide is the term has an emotive meaning of disapproval that we prefer not to apply to certain kinds of ambiguous cases. The very logic of the term therefore tends to prejudice any pending moral analysis of the rightness or wrongness of suicide. As a means to try to deal with this problem they propose an "uncorrupted definition of suicide as what occurs "if and only if one intentionally terminates one's own life--no matter what the conditions or precise nature of the intention or the causal route to death" (Beauchamp, Childress, 1979:87).[3]

As sympathetic as one must feel with their attempt to provide a clear and non-prejudical account of suicide, however, the very idea of an "uncorrupted" definition of suicide distorts the very grammar of such notions. Beauchamp and Childress are quite right to point out that the notion itself cannot settle how and why suicide applies to certain kinds of behavior and not others. But what must be admitted, as Joseph Margolis has recently argued, is the culturally variable character of suicide. There are many competing views.

[3]Elsewhere Beauchamp provides a fuller account arguing suicide occurs when "a person intentionally brings about his or her own death in circumstances where others do not coerce him or her to the action, except in those cases where death is caused by conditions not specifically arranged by the agent for the purpose of bringing about his or her own death" (Beauchamp, 1980:77).

about the meaning and nature of suicide, "some religious, some not, some not even significantly so characterized.... There is no simple formula for designating, except trivially, an act of taking, or yielding, or making likely the end of, one's life that will count, universally as suicide. No, some selection of acts of this minimal sort will, in accord with an interpreting tradition, construe what was done as or as not suicide; and, so judging, the tradition will pro-vide as well for the approval or condemnation of what was done. In short, suicide, like murder itself, is an act that can be specified only in a systematic way within a given tra-dition; and that specification itself depends on classifying the intention of the agent. We can say, therefore, that there is no minimal act of commission or omission that counts as suicide, except relative to some tradition; and, within particular traditions, the justifiability of particular sui-cides may yet be debatable" (1979:25-26).

So the very way one understands "suicide" already in-volves moral judgments and requires argument. So I shall contend that if we rightly understand what life is about, suicide should be understood negatively and should not there-fore be recommended as an alternative for anyone. This is not to deny that from certain perspectives suicide can be considered rational--as an institution, that is a way of characterizing a whole range of behavior, as well as an in-dividual act. That it can be so understood, however, reveals how little the issue turns on the question of "rationality." We must rather ask whether the tradition through which we understand the meaning and nature of suicide is true.

3. WHY SUICIDE IS PROHIBITED

I have argued elsewhere that suicide as an institution must be considered morally doubtful. That conclusion is based on the religious understanding that we should learn to regard our lives as gifts bestowed on us by a gracious Creator (Hauerwas, 1977:101-115). That such an appeal is explicitly religious is undeniable, but I would resist any suggestion that the religious nature of this appeal disqual-ifies it from public argument. Rather it is a reminder of Margolis' contention that any account of suicide necessarily draws on some tradition. Therefore my appeal to this kind of religious presupposition is but an explicit avowal of what any account of suicide must involve--though I certainly would not contend that the only basis for disapproving suicide is religious.

It is important, however, that the significance of the shift to the language of gift be properly appreciated. For it is a challenge to our normal presumptions about the way the prohibition of suicide is grounded in our "natural desire to live." Indeed it is not even clear to me that we have a "natural desire to live," or even if we do what its moral significance entails. The very phrase "natural desire to live" is fraught with ambiguity, but even worse it seems to suggest that when a person finds they no longer have such a desire there is no longer any reason for living.

In contrast the language of gift does not presuppose we have a "natural desire to live," but rather that our living is an obligation. It is an obligation that we at once owe our Creator and one another. For our creaturely status is but a reminder that our existence is not secured by our own power, but rather requires the constant care and trust in others. Our willingness to live in the face of suffering, pain, and sheer boredom of life is morally a service to one another as it is a sign that life can be endured as well as a source for joy and exuberance. Our obligation to sustain our lives even when they are threatened with or require living with a horrible diseases is our way of being faithful to the trust that has sustained us in health and now in illness (Hauerwas, 1979:229-237). We take on a responsibility as sick people. That responsibility is simply to keep on living as it is our way of gesturing to those who care for us that we can be trusted and trust them even in our illness.

There is nothing about this position which entails that we must do everything we can do to keep ourselves alive under all conditions. Christians certainly do not believe that life is inherently sacred and therefore it must be sustained until the bitter end. Indeed the existence of the martyrs are a clear sign that Christians think the value of life can be overriden (Hauerwas, 1980). Indeed I think there is much to be said for distinguishing between preserving life and only prolonging death, but such a distinction does not turn on technical judgments about when we have in fact started dying, though it may involve such a judgment (Hauerwas, 1974:166-186). Rather the distinction is dependent on the inherited wisdom of a community that has some idea of what a "good death" entails (Hauerwas, 1978a:329-336).

Such a death is one that allows us to remember the dead in a morally healthy way--that is, the manner of death does not prevent the living from remembering the manner and good of their life. To be sure we can train ourselves to remember a suicide as if the suicide said nothing about their life, but I think we would be unwise to do so. For to face the reality of a death by suicide is a reminder how often our community fails to offer the trust necessary to sustain our lives in health and illness. Suicide is not first a judgment about the agent, but a reminder that we have failed to embody as a community the comitment not to abandon one another. We fear being a burden for others, but even more to ourselves. Yet it is only by recognizing that in fact we are inescapably a burden that we face the reality and opportunity of living truthfully.

It is just such a commitment that medicine involves and why the physician's commitment to caring for the sick seems so distorted by an ethics of autonomy. Medicine is but a gesture, but an extremely significant gesture of a society, that while we all suffer from a condition that cannot be cured, nonetheless neither will we be abandoned. The task of medicine is to care even when it cannot cure (Hauerwas, 1975:145-150). The refusal to let an attempted suicide die is only our feeble, but real, attempt to remain a community of trust and care through the agency of medicine. Our prohibition and subsequent care of a suicide draws on our profoundest assumptions that each individual's life has a purpose beyond simply being "autonomous."

4. REASONS FOR LIVING AND "RATIONAL SUICIDE:" AN EXAMPLE

However the kind of religious appeals I have made as well as this kind of talk about "purpose" can easily be misleading. For it sounds as though suicide is religiously prohibited because people who believe in God really know what life is about. But that is not the case--at least in the usual sense a phrase such as "what life is about" is understood. Indeed the very reason that living is an obligation is that we are to go on living even though we are far from figuring out what life is about. Our reason for living is not that we are sure about the ultimate meaning of life, but rather because our lives have been touched by another and through that touch we believe we encounter the very being that graciously sustains our existence.

Indeed one of the problems with discussions of "rational suicide" is they seem to be determined by the assumption that the decision to live or to die turns on whether life, and more importantly, one's particular life, has meaning or purpose. Thus, Margolis, for example, suggests that a relatively neutral understanding of the issue raised by suicide is whether the deliberate taking of one's life in order to simply to end it, not instrumentally for any ulterior purpose, can ever be rational or rationally justified. He suggests a rational suicide is when a person "aims overridingly at ending his own life and who, in a relevant sense, performs the act. The manner in which he suicides may be said to be by commission or omission, actively or passively, directly or indirectly, consciously or unconsciously, justifiably or reprehensibly--in accord with the classificatory distinctions of particular traditions" (Margolis, 1975:29). According to Margolis such suicide is more likely to be justified if the person "decided that life was utterly meaningless" or sincerely believed life to have no point at all" (1975:24).

My difficulty with such a suggestion is that I have no idea what it would mean to know that life, and in particularly my life, was "utterly meaningless" or had "no point at all." In order to illustrate my difficulty about these matters let me call your attention to one of the better books about suicide--John Barth's, The Floating Opera.[4] Barth's book consists of Todd Andrews' account of how one day in 1937 he decided to commit suicide. There was no particular

[4]For a similar approach from which I have learned much see Nielsen (1979). The fact that we must resort to example when considering such matters is an important indication how easily abstract discussions of the rightness or wrongness of suicide, for which there is no substitute and must certainly be done, can as easily mislead as they can help us clarify why the suicide is rightly understood in a negative manner. Seldom are any of us sure why it is we act and do not act as we do. We may say we would rather die than live with such and such disease, but how can we be so sure that is the reason. Beauchamp and Childress' suggestion that ideally a person contemplating suicide would consider all the variables is as much a formula for self-deception as one for self-knowledge. I suspect that is why Barth's book is so helpful --namely it is only by telling a story that we come to understand how the prohibition against suicide is meant to shape the self.

reason that Andrews decided to commit suicide and that, we discover, is exactly the reason he decided to do so--namely there is no reason for living or dying.

The protagonist has written the book to explain why he changed his mind and in the process we discover quite a bit about him. Most people would describe him as a cynic, but there is more to him than that. Andrews makes his living by practicing law in a small backwater town in the Cheasapeake tidewater country. He became a lawyer because that is what his father wanted, but he is later stunned by his father's suicide. What bothered him was not that his father killed himself, but that he did so because he could not pay his debts due to the Depression.

Andrews has chosen to live free from any long term commitments since the day in W.W. I when he killed a German sergeant with whom he had shared a foxhole through a terrible night of shelling. His lack of commitment extends even to his arrangement for living--he lives in a hotel room where he registers on a day to day basis. He has, however, been involved in a long term affair with Jane Mack, his best friend's wife. Harrison Mack not only approved but actually arranged this as a further extension of their friendship. However by mutual agreement they have recently decided to end this form of their relation.[5] This is partly the result of the recent birth of Jeannie, who, even though her paternity remains unclear, has given the Macks a new sense of themselves as a couple.

Andrews also suffers from two diseases--subacute bacteriological endocarditis and chronic infection of the prostate. He was told thirty-five years ago that the former could kill him any time. The latter disease only caused him

[5]Andrews admits that this turn of affairs made him reconsider briefly his decision to commit suicide since the Mack's might interpret his suicide as caused by their decision. But he says that this lasted only a moment since it occurred to him "What difference did it make to me how they interpreted my death? Nothing, absolutely, makes any difference. Nothing is ultimately important. And, that, at least partly by my own choosing, that last act would be robbed of its real significance, would be interpreted in every way but the way I intended. This fact once realized, it seemed likely to me that here was a new significance, if possible even more genuine" (1956:224).

to cease living a wastrel's existence he had assumed during law school and begin what he claims is almost a saintly life. And indeed his life is in many ways exemplary, for he is a man who lives his life in accordance with those convictions he thinks most nearly true.

Even though he is not a professional philosopher, Andrews is a person with a definite philosophical bent. For years he has been working on notes, suitably filed in three peach baskets, for the writing of a Humean type Inquiry on the nature of causation. For if Hume was right that causes can only be inferred then his task is to shorten as much as possible the leap between what we see to what we cannot see. That is, to get at the true reasons for our actions.[6]

This becomes particularly relevant if we are to understand Andrews' decision to commit suicide. He fully admits that there are abundant psychological reasons, for those inclined for such explanations, to explain his suicide--a motherless boyhood, his murder of the German sergeant, his father's hanging himself, his isolated adulthood, his ailing heart, his growing sexual impotency, injured vanity, frustrated ambition, boredom--the kinds of things psychoanalysts identify as "real" causes (1956:224). But for him the only reason that interest him in dying are philosophical which he states in five propositions which constitute his completed Inquiry. They simply are:

I. Nothing has intrinsic value. Things assume value only in terms of certain ends.

[6]The full title is actually On Inquiry into the Circumstances Surrounding the Self-Destruction of Thomas F. Andrews, of Cambridge, Maryland, on Ground-Hog Day, 1930 (More Especially into the Causes Therefor). For Andrews tells us his aim is simply to learn why his father hanged himself. Andrews admits the real problem was one of "imperfect communication" between him and his father as he could find no adequate reason for his father's act. His Inquiry, however, became primarily a study of himself since he realized to understand imperfect communicatives requires perfect knowledge of each party. Andrews suggests at the end of the book if we have not understood his change of mind he is again cursed with imperfect communication--but the suggestion seems to be we have a better chance at communication than he had with his father as now at least we have Todd Andrews' story.

II. The reasons for which people attribute value to things are always ultimately arbitrary. That is, the ends in terms of which things assume value are themselves ultimately irrational.
III. There is, therefore, no ultimate 'reason' for valuing anything.
IV. Living is action in some form. There is no reason for action in any form.
V. There is, then, no 'reason' for living (1956:238-243).

And so Todd Andrews decided to kill himself one day in 1937.

However before doing so he decides to go see The Original and Unparalleled Floating Opera, a local minstrel show on a rundown show boat. The absurdity of the show matches perfectly Andrews view of the absurdity of life. During the performance, Andrews goes to the ship's galley, turns on the gas only to be interrupted and saved by a workman who angrily calls him a damn fool--not because he tried to take his life, but because he could have blown up the ship.

More importantly, however, just as he is recovering the Macks, who had also been attending the Opera, rush into the galley with Jeannie who had suddenly taken sick and fainted. Though appealed to for help, Andrews suggests he is no good at such things and advises the Macks to rush to the hospital. However, the local doctor arrives and advises an alcohol rub reassuring everyone nothing is seriously wrong. In the emergency, however, and the concern Andrews felt about Jeannie, he discovers he no longer wants to commit suicide even though he could still easily jump into the Choptank river. For as he tells us, "something was different. Some qualitative change had occurred, instantly, down in the dining room. The fact is I had no reason to be concerned over little Jeannie, and yet my concern for that child was so intense, and had been so immediately forthcoming, that (I understood now) the first desperate sound of Jane's voice had snapped me out of a paralysis which there was no reason to terminate. No reason at all. Moreover, had I not, in abjuring my responsibility for Jeannie, for the first time in my life assumed it--for her, for her parents, and for myself? I was confused, and I refused to die that way. Things needed explaining; abstractions needed to be straightened out. To die now was simply out of the question, though I hated to spoil such a perfect day" (1956:266).

Andrews suspects that most philosophizing to be ration-
alizations but nonetheless his experience requires him to
return to the propositions of his <u>Inquiry</u> to make a small
revision of the fifth:

V. There is, then, no 'reason' for living (or for suicide) (1956:270). For now he tells us that he realized that
even if values are only relative there are still relative
values. "To realize that nothing has absolute value is surely, overwhelming, but if one goes no further from that proposition than to become a saint, a synic, or a suicide on
principle, one hasn't gone far enough. If nothing makes any
final difference, that fact makes no final difference either,
and there is no more reason to commit suicide, say than not
to, in the last analysis. Hamlet's question is, absolutely,
meaningless. A narrow escape" (1956:270).

The Christian prohibition of suicide is clearly based
in our assumption that our lives are not ours to do with as
we please. But that prohibition is but a reminder of the
kind of commitments that make suicide which appears from
certain perspectives and at particular times in our lives so
rational, so wrong. It reminds us how important our commitment to be the kind of people who can care about a sick little girl and in the process learn to care for ourselves.
That kind of lesson may not give life meaning, but it is certainly sufficient to help us muddle through with enough joy
to sustain the important business of living.

REFERENCES

Augustine (1977). "The City of God." Translated by Henry
    Bettenson. Harmondsworth: Penguin.
Barth J (1956). "The Floating Opera." New York: Avon.
Beauchamp T (1980). Suicide. In Regan, T (ed): "Matters of
    Life and Death," New York: Random House, pp. 67-108.
Beauchamp T, Childress J (1979). "Principles of Biomedical
    Ethics." New York: Oxford University Press.
Bergman F (1977). "On Being Free." Notre Dame: University of
    Notre Dame Press.
Dworkin G (1978). Moral Autonomy. In Engelhardt H, Callahan
    D (eds): "Morals, Science, and Sociality," Hastings-on-
    Hudson, New York: Hastings Center Publication, pp. 156-
    171.
Hauerwas, S (1974). "Vision and Virtue." Notre Dame: Fides
    Claretian.

Hauerwas S (1977). "Truthfulness and Tragedy." Notre Dame: University of Notre Dame Press.
Hauerwas S (1978). Care. In Reich W (ed): "Encyclopedia of Bioethics," pp. 145-150.
Hauerwas S (1978a). Religious Conceptions of Brain Death. In Korein, J (ed): "Brain Death: Interrelated Medical and Social Issues," New York: New York Academy of Sciences, pp. 329-338.
Hauerwas S (1979). Reflections on Suffering, Death, and Medicine. Ethics in Science and Medicine 6: 229-237.
Hauerwas S (1980). "Community of Character." Notre Dame: University of Notre Dame Press.
Margolis J (1975). "Negativities: The Limits of Life." Columbus: Merriall.
Nielsen H (1979). Margolis on Rational Suicide: An Argument for Case Studies in Ethics. Ethics, 89, 4: 394-400.
New York Times (1980). British "Right to Die" Group Plans to Publish a Manual on Suicide. p. A18.

Rights and Responsibilities in Modern Medicine: The Second
Volume in a Series on Ethics, Humanism, and Medicine: 201—209

RATIONAL SUICIDE AND MEDICAL ETHICS

Jerome A. Motto, M.D.

University of California School of Medicine

San Francisco

INTRODUCTION

A physician's commitment to preservation of life is
never tested more than when faced with a patient
contemplating suicide. When the suicidal intent is on a
rational basis as a means of relief from intense
psychological pain the dilemma is compounded, as the
traditional medical value of alleviating suffering is in
direct conflict with that of preserving life.

The physician in this situation is confronted with
such questions as, "Why should I go on living?", "What is
the purpose of life--what am I here for?", "I just can't
stand it any more--why not end it?" These are not medical
issues, but theological and philosophical questions that a
traditional medical education does not prepare one for.
Our present task is to propose guidelines for ethical
behavior when presented with this problem in a medical
setting, defining "ethics" as the science of moral values
and duties: the study of ideal human character, actions
and ends.

Suicidal thoughts or impulses are generated when a
person experiences a level of pain exceeding a threshold
that is unique to that individual. The pain may be
physical or emotional in origin, sometimes both, but
usually with a predominant emotional component. The sources
of pain are infinitely varied in different individuals and
can be characterized from a number of perspectives, e.g.,
sociological, psychological, existential or biological.

Whatever the specific situation may be, the term "suicide" refers to a non-coerced, self-inflicted, self-intended death.

The meaning of "rational," as used here in relation to suicide, is that the judgment or decision in question is based on a thorough and realistic assessment of all the available pertinent facts. Such an assessment must thus be carried out before "rational suicide" can be contemplated. The presence of a clear sensorium is not sufficient.

To sharpen our view it is important to specify some further exclusions:
1) We are <u>not</u> considering the "right" to suicide or to prevent suicide. We accept that these rights exist, at least under certain circumstances.
2) We are <u>not</u> including children or adolescents. Society's protective role as regards the young requires separate consideration of these age groups.
3) We are <u>not</u> including persons suffering from delirium, panic states, psychosis or other mental illness which would grossly interfere with the process of forming a reasoned judgment.
4) We are <u>not</u> considering euthanasia. This is a related and sometimes overlapping issue which requires active participation of a second party.
5) We are <u>not</u> using a "terminal illness" model. Contemporary social and legal trends have effectively reduced the level of ethical conflict in this situation.

With the exception of these specific considerations, what constitutes ethical behavior on the physician's part when faced with a patient contemplating rational suicide?

*Throughout this discussion, "hiser" indicates "his and/or her," "heshe" indicates "he and/or she" and "himer" indicates "him and/or her."

ETHICAL RESPONSE TO THE SUICIDAL PATIENT

Our first ethical task is to join with the patient in reviewing all aspects of hiser* life situation, both as to clear perception of the facts and realistic interpretation of the facts. We must acknowledge from the outset that every person's perception is reality to himer and that we all have limited ability in identifying the true meaning of events. Yet whatever skill we have, combined with an empathic "medical attitude," we are obligated to place at the service of our patient. By doing so in a meticulous and compassionate way we assure ourselves that we are aware of all the available pertinent facts and we assure the patient that we understand and respect hiser situation.

The inquiry would include such issues as the compatability of suicide with the patient's prior pattern of approach to problems that seemed insoluble, the possible effect of their suicide on other persons in their life--especially children, what the attitude of prior significant persons would have been (e.g., parents) even though they may now be deceased, what would happen with unfulfilled obligations, projects or goals, is there any conflict with spiritual values, and do they have any fantasies about what would take place in the world as a result of their death.

Having examined all the facts as best we can, our criterion for determining the rationality of the patient's decision is based on our intuitive, subjective judgment, faulty as it may be, as to whether the patient's awareness and assessment of the facts appears realistic to us. We may not agree with the decision, but if it is the best judgment the patient is capable of exercising while in control of hiser reasoning function, we must respect it.

If the patient seems to see all the facts clearly and still opts for suicide, the next step is to assure that all alternatives to suicide are thoroughly explored, including simply temporizing. The direction of the suicidal person's ever-present ambivalence can be shifted by time alone, and delaying the act does not require that the option for suicide be relinquished. The tone of this inquiry is profound respect for the utter finality and irreversibility of suicide, so if other alternatives might be bearable even temporarily, they could reasonably be tried first.

If appropriate resources are available the patient should be asked to discuss hiser thoughts with a person who is especially well acquainted with the suicide issue, or the broader issue of death and dying, on the chance that some benefit might be obtained. The physician, too, would do well to share the situation with a colleague and consultant, preferably one who has special interest and experience with suicidal persons.

With the patient's consent, the circumstances should also be discussed with appropriate family members, minister or other significant persons, to allow some chance for other alternatives to be suggested, and for psychological preparation, leave-taking and mutual support without need for surreptitiousness or isolation. The physician should participate in this to the extent that heshe is able and that the patient requests. If the family is negative about such a plan, time should be taken to let the patient attempt to resolve the issue with them. Family members and friends are free to respond to such situations in ways not open to the physician, whose professional role has stricter limits. The family's alternatives should be made known to them, either by the physician or someone acquainted with the situation.

If the patient does not want the family to know of suicidal plans there is an ethical obligation to inform them nonetheless. Whether this obligation overrides the patient's right to confidentiality can only be decided by the specific circumstances, so a general rule cannot be applied. In any case the patient should be informed of any communication with family members or others.

When the patient asks, "Don't you think this is the best way?" or "What would you do in this situation?", the physician would be most candid to acknowledge that heshe cannot know how the circumstances would be experienced or what alternative chosen if roles were reversed. A useful avenue can be opened, however, by asking the patient how they would answer that question if it were put to them by another person, e.g., family member, friend, patient, client, parishioner, or colleague.

If the patient asks for information about lethal doses, over-the-counter drugs, or possible complications (e.g., vomiting an ingested drug), it would be appropriate to discuss these questions openly and freely. This would necessarily include a statement about the unpredictability of biological resistance and individual differences in drug metabolism. The patient's desire for definition of a lethal instrument for ingestion can realistically be answered by uncertainty as regards medications in common use.

If the patient requests the physician's <u>active</u> collaboration (e.g., prepare a lethal instrument and aid in its use) it would be a moral act to comply if it were consistent with the physician's own philosophy, but would be professionally unethical and a violation of the law as an act of euthanasia. As for <u>passive</u> collaboration (e.g., prescribing an appropriate medication such as digitalis or a sedative, and informing the patient of the effects of overdose), sound ethical justification can be based on the principle of giving the person a choice in the time, place and manner of hiser own death. There is little doubt that such events now occur frequently, but because of lagging social and legal acceptance are not openly acknowledged.

The element of a passive rather than active role for the physician is crucial. We are too aware of the frequency of a last-second reversal of intent in carrying out a suicide plan not to allow that possibility its full potential. For some persons it is only at that moment that the full implication of the act is appreciated. The very presence of a second party, to say nothing of their participation, could weigh in the balance at this critical point and influence what must be an autonomous choice. Only if the final act is under the patient's complete control can we be confident of the non-coercive aspect of the final decision.

The fact that passive collaboration now involves honorable physicians, loving families and grateful patients suggests that socially sanctioned suicide, in some form, is an inevitable development. This prospect is comparable to the status of legal abortion 15-20 years ago, when reputable doctors were joining with the legal and social professions to persuade legislators that society was ready for a change. The reception of Doris Portwood's "Common Sense Suicide: The Final Right" (Portwood 1978), the persistent voice of the clergy, and the recent publication of a booklet in Great Britain to assist would-be suicides

all point to a rising tide of feeling that there is an
acceptable role for suicide, as a form of controlled death,
in our social system.

Even now, the idea of controlled death has been
introduced by an uneasy medical-legal-societal agreement
that in certain cases of terminal illness a life may be
relinquished even though technical means exist to prolong
it. History is replete with suicides that were considered
a more honorable course than available alternatives. It
seems clear that under certain conditions, defined by a
given culture or sub-culture, suicide can have an acceptable
place. It only remains to define what those conditions are.

Individual uniqueness is so great, it is not possible
to formulate specific criteria that will apply to everyone.
What may constitute a rational act in one society may not
be so in another. What may be rational for a person in late
life may not be so for a young adult. For the physician
with a suicidal patient, groping for ethical guidelines,
there is nothing more valid to guide himer as to whether
the patient has come to a rational decision than an
intuitive judgment based on all the information that has
been obtained about that patient. It is most difficult
when the patient is neither mature nor wise, especially
when heshe embraces a philosophy that negates the physician's
own valuing of life.

Reluctance by society to accept this individualized
approach to rational suicide may reflect a persisting taboo
about death, especially if self-inflicted. It can also be
understood on the basis of fearing its indiscriminate or
irresponsible use as well as inflicting a heavy load of
responsibility on the individual physician. A writer on
religious affairs (Cassels 1971) states, "I suspect many
Catholic and Protestant moral theologians would acknowledge
privately that there may be extreme circumstances in which
suicide could be the lesser of two evils. But they would
shrink from saying this publicly, because they feel that
the rule against suicide must be stated as firmly and
inflexibly as possible if it is to serve as a moral prop
for a human being in an hour of desperate despair." If
this statement is correct, perhaps these theologians give
too little credence to Nietzche's point that the thought of
suicide can be a great consolation by means of which one
gets successfully through many a bad night.

Contrary to abortion, in which social acceptance probably increases the incidence, assuring a person the choice of a quick, sure, painless and dignified demise can reduce the suicidal impulse. Dr. Laurens White, a distinguished internist and oncologist, speaks of a patient who, when assured her suicidal goal would not be prevented, decided to continue her life, saying, "The great thing was, once I knew I could do it, life became valuable again. I was back in charge." (White 1971) Some patients express this intense need for a sense of control by a willingness to continue their life only if they have access to a lethal supply of medications.

The very process of exploring the option of rational suicide, as detailed above, can also lead to diminution of the suicidal impulse. Though that is not its primary purpose, the experience of examining one's life in a setting of acceptance and understanding will reduce the pain level in some persons to the point that suicide is no longer an immediate issue. There is relatively infrequent opportunity to observe this in the average physician's office, but it is seen quite often in suicide prevention and crisis facilities.

FURTHER CLINICAL OBSERVATIONS

A physician who had been running an abortion clinic recently joined the anti-abortion movement with the explanation that as he came to see each fetus as a person it became more and more difficult to consider abortion an ethical act. Experience with suicidal patients, on the other hand, suggests that while reverence for life inclines one initially to try to preserve life under any circumstances, one comes to recognize that humane regard for a patient's well-being and dignity sometimes requires acceptance of a decision to relinquish life. To do otherwise is to force the person both to continue an unwanted or agonizing existence and to lose what is most precious to them--their self-respect based on their image of themselves as a functioning, contributing member of society.

A 58-year-old woman faced the amputation of one leg. She told her physician she had considered all the implications of this--the need for a recuperative period, a prosthesis, a rehabilitation program, subsequent limitation of mobility and adaptation to an altered body image. She pointed out that she had come from a rural background, had always retained her love of nature and a vigorous outdoor life, a life that had "kept her going." In the absence of anyone dependent on her, and having accomplished those goals in life that were important to her, she decided she would prefer to end her life at this point and forego the challenge of achieving a new adjustment. She acknowledged that she had the capacity to cope with the change, but simply felt unwilling to do so. She said, "I'm ready to die... this is the right time for me. Some people are afraid of death, but I am not." A careful psychiatric assessment did not reveal anything that would challenge the rationality of her decision. The psychiatrist's recommendation to accede to the patient's wish was accepted and carried out in a dignified, compassionate, passive--and ethical--way.

Percy W. Bridgeman, 1916 Nobel Laureate in physics, wrote in his suicide note, "It isn't decent for society to make a man do this for himself." (deFord 1963) Anyone who works in a coroner's office soon learns what he meant; how lacking in dignity it can be--not to say demeaning, degrading and psychologically brutalizing--to bring about a self-inflicted death in a covert way.

At the same time we shrink from the awful responsibility of examining such life-death decisions on the strength of our intuitive judgment. We want clear rules, some measurement of accuracy, a sense of being in a scientific discipline--in short some assurance that we are doing the right (ethical) thing. Yet we know in our heart of hearts that it is not enough for someone to simply <u>tell</u> us how to do the right thing. If we relinquish trust in our capacity to determine ethical action based on each unique set of circumstances encountered, we give up the most basic value from which ethical action springs, freedom of thought and judgment. That inevitable errors will create distress in the exercise of this judgment is a necessary price of the human experience.

Our moral challenge is to be non-moralizing. Our duty and goal is to help our patients. In considering with them the issue of rational suicide, ethical conduct is best determined not only by what we are told but by the dictates of a humane and caring spirit. It is part of our task as physicians to nurture that spirit and trust its influence on our judgment.

REFERENCES

Cassels L (1971). San Francisco Chronicle, June 5, 1971, p 38.
deFord M (1963). Do we own ourselves? The Realist, June 1963, p 10.
Portwood D (1978). "Commonsense Suicide: The Final Right." New York: Dodd, Mead.
White L (1971). The quality of life. California's Health, Vol. 28-9, p 4.

DISCUSSION SUMMARY: RATIONAL SUICIDE

Marc D. Basson

Director, CEHM
University of Michigan
Ann Arbor, Michigan

Over two-thirds of the discussants felt that many suicides
including the one in this case were both rational and morally
permissible. They tended to justify this intuition by appeal
to utilitarian considerations (decreased or ended suffering
and the elimination of excessive burdens on relatives or
society) and to reject others' paternalistic tendencies.
Those who believed suicide to be morally wrong offered a
number of justifications. Several were convinced by theological arguments such as Hauerwas offered. ("We are made in
God's image and may not destroy that image." "God gave us
life and we have no right to reject it.") Many others were
more concerned with the patient's relationship to his family
and to society. One student commented, "People are political
animals. Your actions impinge on others. You cannot relin-
guish your responsibility to them by giving your own life."
Others suggested that society would be less well off without
the burden of such patients, either because of the spiritual
considerations Hauerwas cites or because there would then be
less stimulus to finds ways to ameliorate or cure the factors
that lead to such suicides. Finally, a few people stated
that a suicide could never be rational and that a would-be
suicide might later "find a new meaning for his life."

Most of those who believed suicide to be sometimes
permissible were prepared to allow the patient in question
to commit suicide but felt that the emergency room physician
was obligated to try to resuscitate him. They also felt that
there was no significant moral difference between active and
passive behavior and so, if legal considerations could be
ignored, were also prepared to attempt to revive him if his

heart stopped so long as they had not had time before the
cardiac arrest to fully evaluate the situation. These people
were also prepared to allow the psychiatrist, after going
through the sort of evaluation that Motto suggests, to give
the patient a prescription for a lethal dose of medication.
Many shrank from the idea of being more active than this in
aiding a suicide for fear of not giving an ambivalent patient
his last chance to change his mind, but most saw no morally
relevant distinction between active aid and passive watching
other than this.

INTRODUCTION: GOVERNMENT FUNDING FOR ELECTIVE ABORTIONS

Marc D. Basson
Director, CEHM
University of Michigan
Ann Arbor, Michigan

Abortion is an emotionally charged subject. When all
is said and done, it seems impossible for proabortionists
and antiabortionists to reach agreement, for the latter
seem to take as a fundamental moral premise that fetuses
have souls and abortion is murder. In many ways, the
situation is like the newer debate over animal rights considered earlier in this volume. Opponents of the status quo
in both cases face a seemingly insoluble problem. How can
one engage in rational moral discourse with a murderer and
persuade him that he is wrong?

The ethical considerations revolving around government
aid to the indigent are equally difficult. What do we owe
the indigent by virtue of their rights? What sort of resource distributions are "fair"? How cost-effective are
the various public policy options? Ought the government to
support an activity which significant numbers of taxpayers
believe to be a serious moral wrong? When we consider
government funding for elective abortions, with all these
issues involved, the debate must inevitably be complex, and
the arguments of our speakers are no exception.

George Sher considers two types of arguments for funding
elective abortions for the indigent, the first based on rights
and the second on utilitarian considerations. He finds
problems with arguments from a right to health care because
it is not clear that elective abortions are, in fact, health
care. Instead Sher seems most impressed with the possibilities of an argument from a general right to welfare, which
would entitle a woman to an abortion along with food and

shelter. Sher describes problems with this sort of argument
as well. General welfare rights of the "have-nots"
inevitably conflict with the property rights of the "haves,"
and their interface is problematic to say the least. However,
Sher seems to believe that such an argument might eventually
be worked out.

He seems more impressed by utilitarian considerations.
Paying for the abortions of indigent mothers maximizes
their liberty, avoids the necessity of government support
for their aborted offspring, and frees both the mother and
the government to concentrate their efforts on already born
children, thus helping them to develop more fully and maximize their potentials. Sher grants that there may be hidden
costs there, such as the possibility of increased disre-
spect for life which the antiabortionists raise, but claims
that on balance utilitarian arguments will probably favor
these abortions.

Sher concludes by considering the unconvinced antiabortionist with fundamentally different moral premises.
The antiabortionist seems impelled by his moral
principles to do anything possible to prevent the murder of
innocent fetuses. Sher feels impelled by his principles to
permit abortions, and in fact probably to fund them with
taxpayers' money.   He urges the development of a higher
order ethical theory about compromise between seemingly irr-
econcilable ethical stances, and suggests that it might be
better for society if both sides would agree on a compromise
that would permit abortion but not fund it and further agree
to limit their opposition to peaceful political protest rather
than firebombing abortion clinics or other violence. The
idea is impressive, but as Sher himself acknowledges it
may be considerably less so to the dedicated antiabortionists.
Suppose the Nazis had promised not to pay for killing Jews
but only to allow the affluent to buy their own guns and
kill Jews privately?

Ann Dudley Goldblatt does not believe that abortion is
morally wrong, but she argues strongly against government
support. She rejects arguments about cost-effectiveness
and keeping down the number of future welfare recipients
as "perverse" and "politically unpalatable". Instead, she
urges two considerations which she believes militate
against federal funding for elective abortions. The first
is a question of eligibility. She points out that the

Medicaid program supports only those who can demonstrate their lack of resources. But, she asks, is not the desperate teenager or the woman whose husband wants a child just as deserving of support? She wonders whether supporting only Medicaid-eligible abortions might not even be considered discriminatory against such psychologically indigent women or against the minorities who might be viewed as being urged to abort their races out of existence. (Goldblatt rejects the option of providing abortions for all as "of staggering costs").

Goldblatt's strongest argument builds on her view of the proper role of medicine. Women need to take responsibility for their own contraception if they intend to be sexually active, Goldblatt argues. She claims that governmental funding of elective abortions would not only directly encourage the indigent to employ abortion as a primary technique but would also seem to convey a societal endorsement of this idea. She rejects the notion that medicine is supposed to compensate for the patient's own refusal to care for herself. Goldblatt would have the government fund elective abortions only for women who had attempted contraception. To charges that this will only encourage women to lie about their previous contraception (or lack there of), Goldblatt replies tartly that in lying the women might at best acknowledge their failure and might be more likely to use proper contraception in the future.

After this conference the Supreme Court voted 5-4 to uphold the Hyde amendment which limits federal support to abortions required to save mothers' lives or in cases of rape or incest. Justice Potter Stewart wrote in the majority opinion that this restriction "places no governmental obstacle in the path of a woman who chooses to terminate her pregnancy, but rather, by means of unequal subsidization of abortion and other medical services encourages alternative activity deemed in the public interest." This departs from the Court's previous decision grounding the right to have an abortion in the right to privacy. Justice William Brennan wrote in the minority decision, "the Hyde amendment's denial of public funds for medically unnecessary abortions" (those which might improve the patient's psychic health but are not lifesaving) "plainly intrudes upon this constitutionally protected decision for both by design and effect it serves to coerce indigent pregnant woman to bear children that they would otherwise elect not to have." The Supreme Court

is the highest Court in the nation and the legality of
restricting abortion funds has been clearly established,
at least for the moment. The ethical questions still
await resolution.

REFERENCES

Harris vs McRae   S.C. #79-1268, June 30, 1978
     (299 Medicare/Medicaid Guide).

Rights and Responsibilities in Modern Medicine: The Second Volume in a Series on Ethics, Humanism, and Medicine: 217—218
© 1981 Alan R. Liss, Inc., 150 Fifth Avenue, New York, NY 10011

GOVERNMENT FUNDING FOR ELECTIVE ABORTIONS

Case for Discussion

"Well, Mrs. Jones, you requested an appointment one month earlier than our usual meeting," said Mrs. McGuire, the social worker for the River Street area.

"You know, Ms. McGuire," said Mrs. Jones, "that I ain't got much money, and with all my bills to pay and the kids, I just had to see you about this new problem."

"What's the matter?"

"I went back to the clinic you told me about, that time for birth control a while back. That doctor, he says I'm pregnant. And I just can't have another one."

"Mrs. Jones, as I look back through your record, I see that you already have four children, and that your husband no longer lives with you and your children."

"Yes, ma'am. Charles took off a year back. But I've been seeing this other fellow now. I just don't know what'll happen if he finds out."

"I see," said Mrs. McGuire. "Now, you've been getting ADC for your children and also welfare."

"You know I got all I can do just to take care of the kids. I just need an abortion, Ma'am."

"Mrs. Jones, I thought you were using birth control, as you said you would when we referred you to the clinic."

"I just couldn't take those pills all the time. I kept forgetting. And that other thing they gave me after my last girl. . ."

"The diaphragm," interrupted Mrs. McGuire.

"Yes, that thing. Well, I just can't seem to use it, and my boyfriend says he didn't like it neither. He said I could always get an abortion."

"Well Mrs. Jones, you know that if you have the child, you'll qualify for more ADC money, and more food stamps. That should help considerably."

"But Mrs. McGuire, I just can't take care of another one. It's just too much."

What is the purpose of programs such as Medicaid? Does society have an obligation to pay for elective abortions such as this one? Why? Or why not? Even if there is no such obligation, should we fund such abortions for prudential reasons, such as the cost to society of unwanted children? Where should the funds come from if such abortions are to be paid for by Medicaid?

Rights and Responsibilities in Modern Medicine: The Second
Volume in a Series on Ethics, Humanism, and Medicine: 219—227
© 1981 Alan R. Liss, Inc., 150 Fifth Avenue, New York, NY 10011

GOVERNMENT FUNDING OF ELECTIVE ABORTIONS

George Sher

University of Vermont

Burlington, Vermont

In this paper, I want to explore some aspects of the
question of whether the government should provide abortions
for women who want but cannot afford them. My method of
approaching this question will be quite straightforward. I
will begin by considering two main arguments in favor of
such funding, and will then go on to discuss some considerations which tell against it. Although the problem obviously
has a legal side as well as a moral one, I shall be concerned only with its moral dimension. Further, my aim will
be not so much to settle the moral issue as to bring out
some main factors pertinent to its resolution.

Whenever one advocates a particular public policy,
there are at least two strategies which he may usefully
employ. He may argue, on the one hand, that the policy
in question is owed to some person or persons as their
right; or he may argue, on the other hand, that the policy
should be adopted because it would tend to promote the
general welfare. We may denominate the first sort of argument an appeal to rights, and the second an appeal to utilities. I shall now consider the degree to which each supports government funding of elective abortions.

Of the two types of argument, it is the appeal to
rights which invokes the weightier sort of moral principle.
When we say that someone has a right to something, we are
not saying merely that it would be nice if he were provided
with it, nor that providing it would be a decent or chari-
table act. Instead, we are saying that there are no two
ways about it--the right-holder must be provided with the

object or service in question. He is entitled to claim it,
and may legitimately complain if his claim is not met
(Feinberg 1970). As Ronald Dworkin has put it, rights are
trumps which take precedence over mere expediency or social
benefit (Dworkin 1977). So if there is a moral right to be
provided with elective abortions, this will constitute a
very strong reason for the government to fund these abortions. But is there in fact such a right?

If one is to show that the right exists, he must answer two distinct questions. The first concerns the right's
derivation. Because a right to be provided with elective
abortions would be extremely specific, it cannot reasonably
be expected to stand alone, independent of all more general
rights. The proposed right, if it exists at all, must be a
derived right; and so our first question is whether there
is a plausible-sounding general right from which it can be
derived. Our second question is how this general right can
itself be grounded and defended.

Given the multitude of plausible-sounding general
rights, we cannot possibly canvass all conceivable sources
of a right to be provided with elective abortions. However,
one leading contender appears to be a general right to be
provided with needed medical care. Abortions, after all,
are performed by medical personnel in a clinical setting,
and involve procedures similar to those employed in other
medical contexts. Yet upon closer inspection, these considerations are far from decisive. First, unlike other
medical procedures, elective abortions are not generally
performed with the aim of improving or maintaining anyone's
health. And, second, the operative fact about medical care
is its role in promoting well-being; and so any right to
medical care would itself seem derivable from a wider right
to the basic prerequisites of well-being. For both reasons,
it is not a right to be provided with medical care, but
rather a right to be provided with the prerequisites of
well-being, which seems the most promising source of a right
to be provided with elective abortions. For ease of reference, we may refer to a right to be supplied with the prerequisites of well-being as a 'general welfare right.

Would a general welfare right support a right to be
provided with elective abortions? In favor of this contention, it can be argued that a child can be a large and continuous drain on a woman's time, energy, and financial

resources. When a woman has as little income as those who would benefit from government funding, such a drain can seriously impair her effective functioning in many areas of life. On the other side, however, it may be replied that the need for abortion is not inevitable like the need for food or shelter, but rather can usually be avoided by taking the proper precautions. Furthermore, any right to the prerequisites for effective functioning might be satisfied by increased government assistance in other areas. Given all of this, the proposed derivation of the right to be provided with elective abortions is at least not obviously correct.

Even if the derivation were unimpeachable, moreover, the problem of grounding and defending a general welfare right would remain. Perhaps the most important difficulty here is that the welfare right would be what is called a positive right. Although it would arise neither from contractual agreements nor from special offices or relationships, it would impose duties which go essentially beyond the duty not to interfere with others. Instead, or in addition, it would impose the obligation to supply the right-holders with particular goods or services under certain conditions. But the only persons who can supply these goods or services are ones who themselves have ownership rights over sufficient wealth or property. Hence, the obligations generated by positive rights are in danger of conflicting with the property rights of others; and if the obligations are backed by sanctions, they are in danger of wrongfully interfering with liberty as well. In view of this, positive rights are essentially more problematical than mere rights of non-interference. (For discussion, see Nozick 1974.)

Although this difficulty is a serious one, it is not necessarily fatal. One way around it would be to deny that property rights are so absolute and all-encompassing that all positive rights must inevitably conflict with them. If property rights were themselves limited--if they required non-interference with a person's property by others under specified conditions only--then they might end where positive rights begin. Of course, no proponent of positive rights has yet produced a powerful general theory which shows that this is the case; but then, neither has any proponent of absolute property rights demonstrated that it is not. Furthermore, there is at least one general theory--the

rational contractor theory of John Rawls (Rawls 1971)--
which might well be adapted to support positive rights.
Although Rawls says very little about rights, he argues
that the correct principles of justice are embodied in certain decisions which would be made by rational individuals
ignorant of their actual positions in life; and he argues
further that these individuals would choose a social system
containing only such inequalities as would work to the advantage of everyone. Within such a system, the institution
of property would exist only insofar as it promoted these
inequalities and no others. Hence, any property rights
that emerged would undoubtedly be hedged with stringent
limitations; and these limitations might well be expressed
in terms of competing positive rights. (For a discussion
of positive rights which makes some contact with Rawls'
position, see Peffer, 1978.)

We can summarize our discussion to this point by
saying that the appeal to rights is potentially weighty
but fraught with difficulties. In view of this, it may be
desirable to turn to a less weighty, but also less problematical, defense of government funding of elective abortions.
This characterization fits the second main argument we will
consider, the appeal to utilities. Generally speaking, a
utilitarian argument is one which justifies an action (or
practice or policy) by appealing to its consequences. The
action, practice, or policy is held to be justified by the
fact that it has better overall consequences--brings more
overall benefit--than any available alternative. It is not
at all clear that we should accept utility as the single
ultimate moral standard; and we have seen that utilities
seem secondary to rights. But even so, it can hardly be
denied that utilitarian considerations are often quite decisive in settling policy questions. As a simple example
of this, consider the regulation of motor vehicle traffic.
Nobody has a moral right to have everyone drive on the same
side of the road, to be given a driving test and license,
or to have speed limits and other regulations enforced.
However, it is obviously very useful for the state to regulate automotive behavior in these ways; and that is quite
sufficient to justify its doing so. What we must now ask
is whether government funding of elective abortions can be
justified in a similar fashion.

At first glance, this suggestion seems to be amply
supported by the benefits promised by such funding. Of

these benefits, one has already been noted. To whatever extent a woman's effective functioning is threatened by her pregnancy, a subsidized abortion benefits her by removing the threat. It allows her to take more effective control of her own life, and to come closer to living the way she wants to live. But beside this, a policy of subsidized abortion has several other major benefits. By providing the services of trained personnel, it reduces the suffering caused by makeshift abortions performed under unsanitary conditions. By limiting competition within the family for attention and money, it enables the recipient's other children to receive more adequate maternal care. And by eliminating the need for society to provide various sorts of further support for infants who would otherwise be born, it frees a substantial amount of society's resources for use in other areas.

Given these considerations, the utilitarian argument for government funding of elective abortions seems a strong one. But like all utilitarian arguments, it rests on a complicated factual claim about the balance of costs and benefits; and this claim may be disputed in its turn. Thus, for example, one might claim that the argument underestimates the benefits of maternity, the benefit of life to the aborted child, or the degree to which subsidized abortion encourages irresponsible decision-making. Or, alternatively, one might maintain that subsidized elective abortion has the extremely harmful effect of eroding respect for all human life--that it is a step down the road to a society in which all unwanted individuals are eliminated. I have my doubts about this last point, partly because any erosion of respect for human life seems more a consequence of the legalization of abortion than its funding. But the truth of the factual claim is less important than the general point it illustrates. If subsidized abortion is to be justified through appeal to its consequences, then we must be sure that all of its consequences, hidden as well as obvious, are given their proper weight.

Even when all of its hidden costs are included, government funding of elective abortions may still be called for on utilitarian grounds. Indeed, I am inclined to believe that this is definitely the case. But even if it is, the question of whether the government should provide such funding remains unsettled; for not all appeals to utility. are equally decisive. We might maximize utility by allowing the police to practice unlimited electronic surveillance and routinely open people's mail. By tolerating these practices, we might imprison many individuals who are a serious menace to society without endangering those who obey the law. But even so, many people would object to these practices on the grounds that they violate a moral right to privacy. And in a parallel way, one might reject the utilitarian defense of government funding of abortion on the grounds that it too violates a moral right, or is seriously wrong in some other way.

As we might expect, the main non-utilitarian objections to government funding of elective abortion are all related to the moral status of abortion itself. To a substantial segment of the population, the zygote or fetus has the same moral standing as a full-grown person, and abortion, whose foreseen result is the death of the zygote or fetus, is therefore tantamount to murder. There are at least three ways in which this belief can be marshalled against government funding for abortions. It might be argued that

(1) Abortion is murder; the government should not finance murder; therefore the government should not finance abortion; or that

(2) Abortion is at least morally dubious; the government should not finance practices which are morally dubious; therefore the government should not finance abortion; or that

(3) Abortion is considered murder by many people; the government should not finance a policy of which many citizens strongly disapprove; therefore the government should not finance abortion.

Of these arguments, the first two focus on our obligations toward the zygote or fetus, while the third focuses on our obligations toward those who oppose abortion. Each argument purports to show that government funding of abortion is unacceptable on non-utilitarian moral grounds. Thus, any one of them, if sound, will weigh against the utilitarian case for government funding.

Do any of the arguments work? The first argument, which says that the government should not provide funding for abortions because abortion is murder, proceeds from a very strong premise. If we agree that abortion is murder, then we must surely also accept the conclusion that the government should not fund it. But precisely because the argument's premise is so strong, it cannot legitimately convince anyone who is not already opposed to all legalized abortion. If someone were to say both that abortion should remain legal and that the government should refuse to fund it because it is murder, he could justly be accused of hypocrisy. He would be espousing one moral standard for the well-off and another for the impoverished. Moreover, what is true of persons here seems true of societies as well. If a society permits the well-to-do to purchase abortions when they want them--as ours does--then it cannot without hypocrisy refuse to fund such abortions for the poor on the grounds that these abortions (and only these?) are murder.

In view of this, the first argument against government funding clearly proves too much. But what, now, of the second argument, which proceeds not from the premise that abortion is murder, but rather from the weaker premise that its moral status is questionable. For this argument, the operative fact is that acute and conscientious thinkers are unable to agree about the status of the fetus--that the principles underlying all positions on the issue seem complex and uncertain. Unlike the stronger premise, this one does not clearly imply that abortion should be illegal. Because it does not, it is not flatly inconsistent to conclude from it that the government should not fund abortion while still maintaining that abortion need not be made illegal. But even if this conclusion is not flatly inconsistent, it is problematical in other ways. For one thing, it may be wondered why the burden of proof should lie on those who view abortion as morally permissible rather than on those who do not. Nor, if the burden does fall on the pro-abortionist, is it obvious why the same moral caution which leads us to withhold funding of abortion should not also lead us to revoke its legality. Failing a convincing rationale for this, the charge that we are applying a double standard will merely reappear in altered guise.

To avoid this charge completely, we must turn to the third argument, which says that the government should withhold funding not because abortion is wrong, but rather because so many people think it is wrong. Although anti-abortionists are just as strongly opposed to the legality of abortion as they are to its funding by the government, it is only its funding which they are forced to support through their own tax dollars. Hence, the argument will not imply that abortion should be illegal if its underlying principle is that citizens should not be forced to pay for practices of which they strongly disapprove. Yet this principle seems unacceptable on other grounds. There is hardly any policy with which some substantial segment of the population does not disagree; and so the principle seems to imply that few if any policies may legitimately be funded with tax dollars. Even if it is modified to apply only to policies to which people object on moral grounds, I suspect that the principle's implications will still be unacceptably extreme.

Given the problems with these three arguments, it is tempting to conclude that as long as elective abortions remain legal, the government should fund them, if only for utilitarian reasons. But before accepting the conclusion, we might briefly consider one further implication of the fact that many people believe abortion to be murder. Given their moral principles, the opponents of abortion must see themselves as obligated to resist abortion relentlessly, through extra-legal means if necessary. On the other hand, given their own moral principles, pro-abortionists must see themselves as committed to resisting such extra-legal tactics in turn. If everyone acts conscientiously, we will face a continuous, no-holds-barred struggle among sincere individuals with incompatible moral principles. Or at least we will face such a struggle if no way of compromising those principles can be found.

I cannot here address all the complexities of moral compromise as it applies to abortion. However, I will end by noting two suggestive facts which emerge from our discussion. The first is that permitting abortions but not funding them--the policy under discussion--incorporates some of what both pro- and anti-abortionists want. The second fact, noted above, is that this policy does not make anti-abortionists pay for abortions, and so avoids forcing them to violate their principles in one especially flagrant way. Given both facts, it seems possible that by leaving elective abortions legal but not funding them, we can achieve a reasonable moral compromise between pro- and anti-abortionists. If we can, then we will have a reason for not funding elective abortions which is far stronger than any yet considered. However, the issues here are deep and complicated, and a detailed discussion of them must be left for another occasion.

REFERENCES

Dworkin R (1977). "Taking Rights Seriously." Cambridge: Harvard.
Feinberg J (1970). The nature and value of rights. J Value Inquiry 4:243.
Nozick R (1974). "Anarchy, State, and Utopia." New York: Basic.
Peffer R (1978). A defense of rights to well-being. Phil & Pub Affairs 8:65.
Rawls J (1971). "A Theory of Justice." Cambridge: Harvard.

Rights and Responsibilities in Modern Medicine: The Second
Volume in a Series on Ethics, Humanism, and Medicine: 229–241
© 1981 Alan R. Liss, Inc., 150 Fifth Avenue, New York, NY 10011

THE FUNDING OF ELECTIVE ABORTION: AN ARGUMENT
OPPOSING JUDICIAL LEGISLATION

Ann Dudley Goldblatt

Division of Social Sciences
The University of Chicago
1126 E. 59th Street, Chicago, Il 60637

My assignment is to defend the proposition that there
should be no government funding of elective abortions. Many
of my colleagues view this as a certainly unsavory and
probably impossible task. Their reasons range from the pragmatic to the principled. In the former category the argument is often blatantly economic: aborting welfare recipients
is cheaper than supporting more welfare recipients. Note here
the assumption that government funding means funding through
public aid, in particular through Medicaid. Those who hold
to this argument most enthusiastically also apparently
assume that an unwanted pregnancy carried successfully to
term by a welfare recipient will be and remain a burden on
society. This seems to me a perverse attitude towards the
potential of a human being, but it is true that in the short
run, aborting costs less than supporting.

The more philosophical arguments frequently focus on
the perception that elective abortion, funded when necessary,
is an essential element of a woman's fundamental liberty to
control her own body.

These examples of arguments favoring the funding of
elective abortions notwithstanding, I believe there are persuasive reasons why federal, state and local governments
should not fund elective abortions. My discussion has three
parts. Part one considers eligibility standards for government funding and the appropriate definition of elective, as
opposed to therapeutic, abortion. Part two asserts that
funding of elective abortions would injure the reputation of
clinical medicine and further encourage the public's neglect

of its responsibility for its health and well-being. Part
three argues that public funding would be politically and
financially infeasible.

PART ONE

I turn now to questions of definition. At first
impression I assumed my topic concerned only elective abortions sought by those eligible to receive Medicaid assistance.
Public funding of all abortions performed on Medicaid
recipients presumably would put categorically and medically
indigent females on a par with other women and adolescent
girls seeking to terminate unwanted pregnancies.

But who is less likely to have the money necessary to
pay for an abortion: the welfare recipient, the fourteen
year old who fears parental censure, the thirty-five year
old wife who fears her husband's response, the rural resident
who can't afford transportation costs, the low income employee
whose health insurance excludes elective abortion? Each may
be equally unable to implement any 'fundamental right' to
decide to terminate her pregnancy.

If government funding were provided through public aid,
whether Medicaid or general public welfare funds, such
funding would be available only to those predetermined to
be categorically or medically needy. Such a policy would
be vulnerable to attack from two directions. First because
it could be perceived as a form of direct discrimination.
Minority women have double the abortion rate, the number
of abortions per 1000 live births, of non-minority women.
Minority women are disproportionately dependent on Medicaid
for medical treatment; 40% of black and other non-white
women are Medicaid-eligible compared to approximately 8% of
white women. (Beal v. Doe, 1977) Given these figures, if
one argues that funding elective abortion is an inducement
to terminate a pregnancy, then public funding may be perceived as government sponsored genocide. Similar arguments
have been made with reference to pre-marital sickle cell
anemia testing, to public aid programs advocating contraception and distributing contraceptives to unmarried adolescents,
and to questionably voluntary welfare recipient sterilizations.

A reverse discrimination can also be argued. Public
welfare funding of elective abortions does not equally protect unemancipated but not Medicaid eligible adolescent

girls, or perhaps all women not categorically or medically needy but nonetheless without the money needed to purchase an abortion.

Government could fund all elective abortions. There could be a statutory claim on public funds vested by the condition of unwanted pregnancy. This could be a program similar to the Maintenance Hemodialysis program. It would be prohibitively expensive, undoubtedly much more expensive than the gloomiest of cost predictions. Consider the hemodialysis program, where the original cost estimates were based on careful projections of the original estimates as to the cost of the hemodialysis program and projected a billion dollar per year cost at the year 2000. Actual annual cost exceeded this figure in 1978, five years after the initiation of the program. (Cummings, 1978)

There is no way to estimate accurately the demand for funded elective abortions. The contraceptive ratio, the amount of contraceptive materials and devices prescribed and sold per 1000 'fertile' women has decreased since the 1973 decisions; the repeat abortion rate, which is admittedly inaccurately low because of a documented tendency to deny previous abortions, has risen faster than original estimates. (Nat.Acad.Sci., 1975) There are indications that abortion has become the birth control measure of choice for many women, not just for minority women on welfare as Justice Marshall concluded in 1977. (Beal v. Doe, 1977)

Until recently any implication that the cost of programs related to health care could be excessive was received with outrage. But we are becoming aware that the public purse is not bottomless, that limitations are unavoidable even for allocations relating to medical care. Where on this list of priorities should we put elective abortion? First we must define elective abortion.

I begin with the January 1980 decision in McRae v. Harris. This decision, written by Judge Dooling of the Eastern District of New York, contains an extensive discussion of what abortions ought to be considered 'medically indicated.' It is to be noted that Judge Dooling avoids discussing what abortions are medically necessary, although the relevant statutory term in the Medicaid statute is 'necessary medical care.'

Judge Dooling argues that each abortion a physician considers appropriate to <u>preserve</u> a woman's state of health is medically indicated, that is, is a therapeutic abortion for which New York Medicaid funds must be made available to reimburse the physician performing the abortion. Judge Dooling argues that every abortion obtained or requested by a Medicaid-eligible woman ought to be considered therapeutic. While pregnancy is not called a disease, it is considered a health endangering condition. In Judge Dooling's words, a pregnant woman must 'assume the risks' of pregnancy through-out her pregnancy. Judge Dooling also questions the state's legitimate power to limit abortions during the third trimes-ter of pregnancy by asserting, that if, at any time during pregnancy, the prenant woman is no longer willing to assume the risks of pregnancy, a requested abortion should be con-sidered a request for a therapeutic abortion.

These conclusions are in opposition to public opinion. A New York Times - CBS poll reported that abortions requested for social, personal, familial or financial reasons are believed to be elective, not therapeutic, abortions. The poll additionally reported that 85% of the persons polled opposed government funding of elective abortions thus defined. (<u>McRae v. Harris</u>, 1980)

I find this definition of elective abortion acceptable. I realize it does not consider the psycho-social aspects of an unwanted pregnancy which may affect a pregnant woman's mental health. But the state of the art of psychiatric diagnosis and prediction is so uncertain and the psychiatric training of non-psychiatrist physicians so limited, that to include all potential mental health sequelae would make any definition of 'elective abortion' meaningless.

Before I turn to part two, let me review my discussion so far. First, I have concluded that it is unclear what persons should or must be eligible to receive public funding for elective abortions. Second, a realistic definition of elective abortion is essential. Finally, a large majority of our population does make a distinction between therapeutic and elective abortions and between privately and publicly funded abortions, and is opposed to government funding of elective abortions.

PART TWO

In this second part of my discussion, I argue that public funding of elective abortion would be wrong because it would distort further the public's perception of the purpose and appropriate use of clinical medicine and would encourage a perception of non-responsibility for individual health and well-being. Government funding would reinforce a growing inclination to see unintentional pregnancy as a disease and abortion its appropriate and necessary medical cure.

I start, as I think I must, by acknowledging that an unwanted pregnancy is an affront and a threat. It shows a lack of control over the biological processes of one's body. It threatens one's image of one's personal future. An unwanted, and particularly an extra-marital or pre-marital pregnancy may also involve social disapproval, a demonstration of promiscuity.

Until recently, and perhaps even today, pregnancy and childbirth were often considered at once the only justification and the proper punishment for a woman's engaging in sexual intercourse. Some of the most intense attacks on this perception have come from the federal judiciary.

The United States Supreme Court, first in Griswold v. Connecticut, a contraception case involving married couples, and more dramatically in Eisenstadt v. Baird, a 1972 decision invalidating statute that prohibited the distribution or sale of contraceptives to unmarried women, attempted to separate totally the exercise of sexuality from the possibility of procreation. This attempted denial of biological cause and effect has created misperceptions, particularly concerning obligations that ought to be inherent in the responsible exercise of sexuality.

A more contemporary assessment of sexuality sees spontaneity as essential to healthy, and particularly to 'modern' sexuality. A study of legal abortions in Hawaii found that 94% of women with unwanted pregnancies expected to engage in sexual intercourse when conception took place. Yet more than half of these women did not use contraceptives, and 80% of this group said they did not use contraceptives because they did not want intercourse to appear planned. This desire for pseudo-spontaneity apparently is designed to misinform the woman's partner as to the expectedness of intercourse and also is an attempt at self-delusion based on a wish to convince the woman herself that intercourse is the result of spontaneous, uncontrollable desire. (Diamond, 1973)

My point is that planned non-marital intercourse, whether or not contraception is used, seems to be morally reprehensible in these women's minds. If intercourse is 'unintentional', a resulting pregnancy is more easily seen as an involuntary, morally neutral medical condition, perhaps even a disease. Abortion then becomes a medical treatment. This perception of pregnancy provided the foundation for the claim of the dissenting justices in the 1977 Supreme Court Medicaid abortion cases that 'stripped' of its moral implications, **abortion and childbirth are 'simply two alternative medical** methods of dealing with pregnancy.' (Maher v. Roe, 1977) Unless both abortion and childbirth are perceived as, and only as, emptyings of the womb, this statement is false. Childbirth is the natural completion of a biological process; abortion is the artificial, premature termination of a natural process.

An important effect of a separation between intercourse and pregnancy is the concurrent perception of abortion as a typical medical treatment. A patient-requested abortion is not a typical example of clinical medical care. A patient-requested abortion presents a patient-diagnosed 'medical' condition together with a demand for a specific patient-pre-scribed treatment. A perceived need for abortion depends on the patient's view of this particular pregnancy as unwanted. We don't speak of unplanned tumors or unwanted gallstones. There are no free standing clinics offering to perform only patient-requested appendectomies.

Most abortions are not performed by the patient's attending or regular physician, assuming she has one. 80% of the abortions performed in Illinois are performed in free-standing for-profit clinics. (Chicago Sun-Times, 1978) These clinics offer no services other than abortions, sterilizations and, in some instances, pregnancy tests of dubious validity.

The etiology of most diseases and pathological conditions is complex, often incomplete and frequently unknown. Pregnancy has a single, known cause. Disease prevention is often uncertain, but the correct use of the most common contraceptives provides from 93 to 99% protection. Pregnancy is repeatable over an average of approximately 30 years. There are instances of women obtaining three and four abortions within one calendar year, and over half of all repeat abortions result from uncontracepted intercourse. (Nat. Acad. Sci., 1975)

For these reasons, and others, elective abortion is an atypical health care service. But even so, why would government funding of this atypical medically mediated service injure the profession of clinical medicine? Because it would encourage the public to view the physician not as a knower-teacher or as a diagnostician and healer but as a plumber of the body, a means to the patient's specific, self-determined end.

The clinical physician's reputation is already in trouble. Forget malpractice, the diet doctors and Dr. Feelgoods. Go to any bookstore. It used to be "Men in White" and "The Microbe Hunters", stories of heroes fighting against death, disease and suffering. Now it's most likely "Coma", "The Terminal Man" and "Heartsounds." This is the physician as villain, profiteer, unscrupulous scientist or as merely careless and uncaring. To too many people, Dr. Jekyll has turned into Dr. Hyde. At the same time, patients are becoming chic consumers, demanding abortions, psychotropic medications and specific diagnostic or surgical procedures. Government funding of elective abortions would help validate the trend towards perceiving the demanding patient and passive physician as the norm of the medical relation. While there are those who find this a healthy trend, I disagree. I think the demanding patient is over-medicated and over-treated, and that the result is bad for our wallets but even worse for our health.

A government policy supporting elective abortion by funding it would also be detrimental to our self-image as responsible, autonomous individuals. The sick role has always had compensating features, particularly the feeling of blamelessness. Most of us are uncomfortable with even the most basic dictates of preventive medicine. We all know smoking, obesity, lack of exercise, bad nutritional habits, too little or too much sleep, too much to drink, and non-compliance with distracting or inconvenient medical regimens affect our health adversely, but few of us control these unhealthy but comforting habits.

Elective abortion is a medically mediated procedure. One of the most attractive attributes of seeing elective abortion as a medical procedure is precisely its association with the blamelessness of illness. But the relation between uncontracepted intercourse and pregnancy is much more direct than that of the unhealthy habits mentioned above and specific diseases or general conditions of ill health. It is immediate, exclusive and almost always preventable.

Government funding of elective abortions would reinforce the seductive image of elective abortion as a medical response to a blameless condition of ill health. This would be a poorly informed policy by itself, to say nothing of its implications with regard to other principles of health maintenance and disease prevention equally difficult to accept as individual responsibilites.

Why is it I would treat the head injuries of the motorcyclist who refused to wear a helmet, but would deny elective abortions? For one reason, because of the degree of likelihood that the situation will be repeated. For another, because the head trauma is an acute life threatening medical emergency. The differences are matters of degree, matters of a potential change in personal health habits, matters of personal and societal responsibilities.

Why not then pay for elective abortions out of welfare funds, as a policy of free choice rather than of subsidized medical care? Such a policy would clearly be, as they say, cost-effective. But the underlying rationale for this policy is politically unpalatable: that it is a good investment because it will reduce the welfare rolls and that the poor should be encouraged to have fewer children.

PART THREE

I turn now to the final part of my discussion. I want to make two more points. First, that government funding would be a government policy favoring elective abortion as a recommended form of family planning. My argument is intended to counter the frequent claim that funding elective abortion would be a neutral response to the constitutional invalidation of prohibiting and restrictive abortion statutes. My second point is that there is strong public opposition to a government policy endorsing elective abortion. Even if the brightest and best of our elected or appointed lawmakers were in favor of funding, it would be imprudent, even if it were possible, to enact such a policy.

Justice Brennan, dissenting in one of the 1977 Medicaid abortion decisions, argues that funding childbirth but not elective abortion unjustly induces poor women to carry pregnancies to term that would not be continued if <u>both</u> childbirth and abortions were funded or if <u>neither</u> were funded. (Maher, 1977) The funding of childbirth and not of elective abortion, however, underscores a legitimate government interest in the safe birth of its citizens. Without citizens, there can be no government. Government can not remain neutral with regard to its infant morbidity and mortality rates.

But is the funding of both childbirth and elective abortion not then simply an equal interest in the health of present and nascent citizens? I don't think so and I don't believe it would be perceived as an equal or a neutral position by the public.

To much of our citizenry, government is in a quite real way a parens patriae. Subsidized elective abortion would represent not merely its legality but its legitimacy. Justice Blackmun's majority opinions in <u>Roe v. Wade</u> and <u>Doe v. Bolton</u> include exhaustive attempts to make abortion a socially and morally appropriate, as well as a legal, response to unwanted pregnancy. But given the resulting polarization of attitudes for and against abortion, Justice Blackmun's attempts were unsuccessful except to the already convinced.

Abortions, while legal, have remained a shadowed, suspect medical treatment. Women frequently deny previous abortions. Too few women seek an abortion or advice concerning where to obtain a safe abortion from their regular physicians. Far too few women have been willing to report painful, septic, incomplete or unnecessary abortion procedures. In contradiction to the cliche of the patient boring others with the story of his or her operation, abortion remains a hidden medical experience.

Legality has done little to change this attitude. The Hyde amendments and the anti-elective abortion statutes and regulations of many state legislatures show that funding of elective abortions is not a viable legislative proposal in most of our states. Assuming the accuracy of public opinion polls, a direct referendum would overwhelmingly oppose government funding of elective abortions. The one way funding of elective abortions could be enforced, and then only for medically or categorically indigent, is by judicial legislation.

Many federal court decisions involving question of
Medicaid-funded abortions have adopted expansive definitions
of what abortions should be paid for under state Medicaid
statutes. Of course, federal and state legislative enact-
ments can be amended or repealed. If a finally authoritative
judicial interpretation of what abortions are medically
necessary is felt to be too inclusive, federal and state
legislatures could redescribe childbirth, prenatal and peri-
natal care as pediatric medical services. Medicaid would
then not cover pregnancy terminations except for those
pregnancies which are life endangering.

The Supreme Court is about to hear oral argument in
several Medicaid abortion cases, including McRae v. Harris,
the case decided by Judge Dooling. I can't predict how the
Court, especially this Court will rule.* But I believe the
Court ought not to adopt a rule holding that the unwantedness
of a welfare recipient's pregnancy is itself sufficient
indication that the requested abortion is medically
necessary to preserve the pregnant woman's health. The Court
should not rule so to impose such a large increment in fiscal burden on federal and state programs already in
severe financial difficulty.

The limitations of the annual Hyde amendments notwithstanding, federal appropriations for Title XIX, the Medicaid
statute, are barely adequate. The need, and the desire, for
medical care is difficult to predict and seemingly impossible
to control. Nowhere is this more apparent than in the case
of elective abortion. Private insurance companies offer
health insurance coverage for abortion but only at high rates
or in experience rated group policies. Many individual
insurance policies limit abortion coverage to inpatient
therapeutic abortions, therapeutic being expressly and
narrowly defined.

Putting fiscal considerations aside, along with the
constitutional spectre of poverty as a sufficient ground for

---

*Judge Dooling's opinion was reversed on June 30, 1980. Harris
v. McRae, 48 U.S.L.W. 4941 (1980) Both the Hyde amendments and
state restrictions on reimbursing for elective abortions
were upheld.

finding a violation of equal protection, the Supreme Court
would act imprudently if it chose to re-enter the abortion
controversy in an activist role. It has become apparent
that the Court was unsuccessful in its attempt to create a
consensus favoring an individual's freedom to choose to
abort her pregnancy. The 1973 Supreme Court's unsophisticated
view of abortion as 'primarily and inherently' a medical
decision to be performed when medically indicated in the
best clinical judgment of the woman's attending physician is
simply untenable. (Roe v. Wade, 1973)

There are indications in the 1976, 1977 and 1979 Supreme
Court abortion decisions that a majority of its justices will
not reiterate the medical-legal fiction that a typical,
traditional doctor-patient relation obtains in the patient-
requested abortion situation. Seen in the light of a typical
abortion clinic experience, this image does make the law
seem an ass and the physician a profit-hungry scalpel for
hire.

The Court need not affirm the expansive rule proposed by
Judge Dooling. It can uphold or strike the Hyde amendments
and still conclude that they do not affect the individual
requirements of state medicaid statutes. It can follow the
1977 Medical abortion precedents and permit some state
regulation of therapeutic abortions as indicative of
legitimate state policies protective of potential life. Or
it can uphold state limitations as an appropriate containment of health care costs to costs of necessary medical
treatment.

In short, and to conclude, funding of elective abortions
by means of judicial 'interpretation', or, more accurately,
judicial legislation, is possible, but would be imprudent.
On the other hand, legislative or popular action requiring the
funding of elective abortions are not viable possibilities.

CODA

The organizers of this conference asked me to comment
briefly on the case of Mrs. Jones. I am obligated by my
arguments above to oppose Mrs. Jones's abortion request. My
reasons, in addition to the constitutional, legal, political
and theoretical reasons already mentioned, are as follows:

The first is awkwardly Macchiavellian. While the number

of Medicaid reimbursed abortions has declined substantially wherever state limitations on reimbursable abortions have been upheld, the number of legal abortions performed has continued to rise and the national birthrate, in particular the birth rate for the indigent segment of the population, has remained stable or declined. Many women in Mrs. Jones's position have apparently obtained the money needed to pay for their abortions from non-public sources.

Secondly, reimbursing Mrs. Jones, or rather the physician who aborts her, would reinforce Mrs. Jones's feeling that the pill is too hard to remember and the diaphragm too much trouble and too intrusive. It would encourage Mrs. Jones's sense of non-responsibility for the normal, expectable consequences of intercourse. It would also encourage a sense of non-control over one's life and its happenings. Thus I would, in many senses reluctantly, deny Mrs. Jones's request.

I find myself obliged to add a hypothetical limitation to my conclusion. If Mrs. Jones had been able to use a diaphragm or oral contraceptive medication and had become pregnant due to contraceptive afilure, then I would argue in favor of funding her abortion. This is consistent with what I believe is the essential argument on behalf of personal responsibility for one's actions to the best of one's ability. I recognize that this position is open to attack as an encouragement to lie about the use of contra-ception. But it seems to me that, even so, to acknowledge what one could have done and ought to have done is better than pretending one had no responsibility at all.

REFERENCES

Beal v. Doe (1977). 432 U.S. 438.
Chicago Sun-Times (1978). December 2, p4, col. 4
Cummings NB (1978). "Federal Funding of Kidney and Urinary Tract Research." Government Printing Office, pp. 244-54
Diamond M, Steinhoff PG, Palmore JA, Smith RG (1973) Sexuality, birth control and abortion: Decision making sequence. J Biosoc Sci 5: 347-61.
Doe v. Bolton (1973). 410 U.S. 179.
Eisenstadt v. Baird (1972). 405 U.S. 438.
Griswold v. Connecticut (1965). 381 U.S. 479.
Maher v. Roe (1977). 432 U.S. 464
McRae v. Harris (1980). 1980 CCH Medicare and Medicaid

Transfer Binder Para. 30, 155; reversed sub nom.
Harris v. McRae (1980). 48 U.S.L.W. 4941.
National Academy of Sciences (1975). "Legalized Abortion and
the Public Health." Washington DC, pp 8-9, 115-23.
Roe v. Wade (1973). 410 U.S.113.

DISCUSSION SUMMARY: GOVERNMENT FUNDING FOR ELECTIVE ABORTIONS

Marc D. Basson
Director, CEHM
University of Michigan
Ann Arbor, Michigan

Seventy percent of the discussants favored federal
funding for abortion, forty five percent for deontological
reasons and the other twenty five percent because of
utilitarian and prudential considerations. The forty five
percent who argued from the rights of the poor seemed most
concerned with the social inequities implicit in restricting
abortions to those who can afford them. Some argued that
an abortion is just like any other aspect of medical care,
aimed at enhancing the patient's welfare and ability to
function in society. Others were prepared to concede that
elective abortions might aim at different goals than much
of the rest of medical practice. Nevertheless, they argued
that every woman should have a right to control her own
body. They felt that this was as fundamental as a right to
food, clothing or education and ought to be guaranteed all
women. The other twenty five percent argued from considerations of cost-effectiveness (the additional cost of
supporting and educating the unaborted child), the un-
happiness of an unwanted child and the mother forced to
bear and raise it, and the possible complications of
illegal abortions.

Those who objected to government funding for abortion
responded that the money would be better spent educating
the indigent to the need for contraception and supplying
it to them. If a woman wants to control her life, they
argued, she should start before she gets pregnant, not
after. They did not perceive a right to have abortions
provided for one and found the analogy to other sorts of
medical care unpersuasive.

SELECTED REFERENCES

FOURTH CONFERENCE

The Right to Health Care

Blackstone, WT (1976). On health care as a legal right:
    Philosophical justifications, political activity, and
    adequate health care. Georgia Law Review 10(Winter):
    391.
Crawford R (1978). You are dangerous to your health. Social
    Policy 7(4):11.
Engelhardt HT, Jr (ed) (1979). "Rights to Health Care."
    J Med Phil 4(2).
Feinberg J (1970). The nature and value of rights. J Value
    Inquiry 4(Winter):243.
Kass L (1975). Regarding the end of medicine and the pur-
    suit of health. Public Interest 40(Summer):11.
Millis JJ (1970). Wisdom? Health? Can society guarantee
    them? NEJM 283:260.
Sade RM (1971). Medical care as a right: A refutation.
    NEJM 285:1288.
Soble A (1976). On health care as a right: More on the
    right to health care. Georgia Law Review 10(Winter):
    525.
Telfer E (1976). Justice, welfare and health care. J Med
    Ethics 2(Sept):107.

Life and Death Decisions in the Neonatal Intensive Care Unit

Duff RS, Cambell AGM (1973). Moral and ethical dilemmas in
    the special care nursery. NEJM 289:890.
Fletcher J (1975). Abortion, euthanasia, and a case of
    defective newborns. NEJM 292:75.
Hare RM (1973). Survival of the weakest. In Gorovitz S (ed):
    "Moral Problems in Medicine." New Jersey: Prentice-
    Hall, p 364.
Jonsen AR, Lister G (1978). Newborn intensive care: The
    ethical problems. Hastings Center Report 6(1):15.
Parfit D (1973). Rights, interests and possible people.
    In Gorovitz (ed): "Moral Problems in Medicine."
    New Jersey: Prentice-Hall, p 369.

Pomerance JJ, Ukrainski CT, Ukra T, Henderson H, Nash AH, Meredith JL (1978). Cost of living for infants weighing 1,000 grams or less at birth. Pediatrics 61(6):908.

Shaw AM, Shaw IA (1973). Dilemmas of "informed consent" in children. NEJM 287:885.

Tooley ME (1972). Abortion and infanticide. Philosophy and Public Affairs 2(Fall):357.

Animal Rights and Animal Experimentation

Baxter DW, Aszewski J (1960). Congenital universal insensitivity to pain. Brain 83:381.

Ethics (1978). 88(Jan):95-178. Papers by Fox, Haworth, Regan, and Singer on "Animal Liberation."

Feinberg J (1974). The rights of animals and unborn generations. Reprinted in: Mappes TA, Zembaty JS (eds) "Social Ethics." New York: McGraw-Hill, p 350.

Regan T (1975). The moral basis for vegetarianism. Can J Phil 5(Oct):181.

Singer P (1975). "Animal Liberation." New York: Random House.

Visscher MB (1972). The newer antivivisectionists. Proc Am Phil Soc 116:157.

Informed Consent

Alfidi RJ (1971). Informed consent: a study of patient reaction. JAMA 216:1325.

Chayet NL (1976). Informed consent of the mentally disabled: A failing fiction. Psychiatric Annals 6(June):82ff.

Cobbs v. Grant, 8 Cal 3d 229, 502, p.2d 1, 104 Cal Rptr 505 (1972).

Freedman B (1975). A moral theory of informed consent. Hastings Center Report 5(4):32.

Fries JF, Loftus EF (1979). Right or rite? CA - A Cancer Journal for Physicians 29(5):316.

Laforet EG (1976). The fiction of informed consent. JAMA 235:1579.

Roth LH, Meisel A, Lidz CW (1977). Tests of competency to consent to treatment. Am J Pysch 134(March):279.

Wilkinson v. Vesey, 295 Atlantic 2nd, p.676.

Woodward WE (1979). Informed consent of volunteers: A direct measure of comprehension and retention of information. Clin Res 27:248.

FIFTH CONFERENCE

The Refusal to Sterilize

Beauchamp TL (1977). Paternalism and bio-behavioral control. The Monist 60(1):62.
Brody H (1976). The physician-patient contract: Legal and ethical aspects. J Legal Med 4(7):25.
Cassell EJ (1976). "The Healer's Art: A New Approach to the Doctor-Patient Relationship." Philadelphia: J.B. Lippincott Co.
Dworkin G (1972). Paternalism. The Monist 56(1):64.
Feinberg J (1971). Legal paternalism. Can J Phil 1:105.
Fried C (1976). Equality and rights in medical care. Hastings Center Report 6(1):29.
Hart HLA (1963). "Law, Liberty and Morality." Stanford: Stanford University Press.
Holder AR (1973). Voluntary sterilization. JAMA 225:1743.
Kao CCL (1976). Maturity and paternalism in health care. Ethics in Science and Medicine 3:179.
Marsh FH (1977). An ethical approach to paternalism in the physician-patient relationship. Ethics in Science and Medicine 4:135.
McGarrah RE Jr., Peck SL (1974). Voluntary female sterilization. Hastings Center Report 4(3):5.
Pasnau RO, Gitlin MJ (1980). Psychological reactions to sterilization procedures. Psychosomatics 21(1):10.
Simonaitis J (1973). The right to sterilization. JAMA 226:1151.
Veatch RM (1974). Sterilization: Its socio-cultural and ethical determinants. In Schima ME (ed): "Advances in Voluntary Sterilization." New York: Elsevier, p 305.
Winston RML (1977). Why 103 women asked for reversal of sterilization. Brit Med J 30:305.

Cost Effectiveness and Patient Welfare

Bayles MD (1978). The price of life. Ethics 89(Oct):20.
Card WI, Mooney GH (1977). What is the monetary value of a human life? Brit Med J 2:1627.
Cleverly W (1977). Cost containment in the health care industry. Topics in Health Care Financing 3(Spring):1.
Fein R (1976). On measuring economic benefits of health programs. In Veatch RM, Branson R (eds): "Ethics and Health Policy." Cambridge: Ballinger Pub Co, p 262.

Fried C (1976). Equality and rights in medical care. Hastings
    Center Report 6(1):29.
Gilson S (1977). Is cost the physician's business? NEJM 296:
    1071.
Havighurst CC (1977). Health care cost-containment regulation:
    Prospects and an alternative. Am J of Law and Med 3:309.
Henley K (1977). The value of individuals. Philosophy and
    Phenomenological Research 37:345.
Jones-Lee MW (1976). "The Value of Life." Chicago: University
    of Chicago Press.
Kaplan MA (1978). What is a life worth? Ethics 89(1):58.
Kassirer JP, Pauker SG (1978). Should diagnostic testing be
    regulated? NEJM 299:947.
Mooney GH (1977). "The Valuation of Human Life." London:
    MacMillan.
Mechanic D (1978). Approaches to controlling the cost of
    medical care: Short-range alternatives. NEJM 298:249.
Neuhauser D, Lewicki AM (1975). What do we gain from the
    sixth stool guaiac? NEJM 222:226.
NEJM 293 (July 31, 1975). Includes papers by McNeil BJ;
    Hiatt HM; Fried C.
Thompson JD, Fetter RB, Shin Y (1978). One strategy for con-
    trolling costs of university teaching hospitals. J Med
    Ed 53(March):167.
"Valuing Lives." Symposium in Law and Contemporary Problems,
    Vol 40(Autumn 1976). Includes papers by Acton, Zeckhauser,
    and Shepard.
Weinstein MC, Stason WB (1977). Foundations of cost-effective-
    ness analysis for health and medical practices. NEJM
    296:716.

The Rational Suicide

Andreasen NJC (1974). Ariel's flight: the death of Sylvia
    Plath. JAMA 228:595.
Motto J (1972). The right to suicide: A psychiatrist's view.
    Life-Threatening Behavior 2(3):183.
Perlin S (1975). "A Handbook for the Study of Suicide." New
    York: Oxford University Press.
Portwood D (1978). "Common Sense Suicide: The Final Right."
    New York: Dodd, Mead and Co.
Pretzel PW (1968). Philosophical and ethical considerations
    of suicide prevention. Bulletin of Suicidology July:30.
Rosen DH (1976). The serious suicide attempt: Five-year
    follow-up study of 886 patients. JAMA 235:1205.

Shneidman ES, Farberow NL, Litman RE (1970). "The Psychology of Suicide." New York: Jason Aronson.

Slater E (1976). Assisted suicide: Some ethical considerations. Intl J of Health Services 6:321.

Szasz TS (1971) The ethics of suicide. The Antioch Review 31:7.

Government Funding for Elective Abortions

Beal v. Doe. 423 US 438 (1977).

Blaumer MA (1976). Medicaid and the abortion right. George Washington Law Review 44:404.

Bryant MD (1976). State legislation on abortion after Roe vs. Wade: Selected constitutional issues. Am J of Law and Med 2(Summer):101.

Butler PA (1977). Right to medicaid payment for abortion. Hastings Law Journal 28(March):931.

Christianity and Crisis (1977). Installments of a debate on religious ethics and medicaid abortion in Sept 19, Oct 3, Oct 31, Nov 14, Dec 26 issues.

Harris v. McRae. S.C. case #79-1268, June 30, 1978 (299 Medicare/Medicaid Guide).

Institute of Medicine (1975). "Legalized Abortion and the Public Health." Washington DC: National Academy of Sciences.

Mahler v. Roe. 423 US 464 (1977).

Petitti DB, Cates WJ (1977). Restricting medicaid funds for abortions: Projection of excess mortality for women of childbearing age. Am J of Publ Heath 67:860.

Roe v. Wade. 93 Sup Ct 705 (1973).

Thomson J (1971). A defense of abortion. Philosophy and Public Affairs 1(1):47.

Unger ZM (1976). Medicaid assistance for elective abortions: The statutory and constitutional issues. St. John's Law Review 50:751.

Author Index

Subject Index